FAO Food and Nutrition Series

No. 11 Rev. 1

HUMAN NUTRITION
IN TROPICAL AFRICA

A textbook for health workers

with special reference to community health problems

in East Africa

by

M.C. LATHAM, O.B.E.

Professor of International Nutrition, Cornell University,
Ithaca, New York, USA

FOOD AND AGRICULTURE ORGANIZATION OF THE UNITED NATIONS
Rome 1979

First edition 1965
Eighth printing 1978
Second edition 1979

This edition has been financed by the Swedish International Development Authority. The first edition was financed by the United Nations Children's Fund under a project jointly sponsored by the Food and Agriculture Organization of the United Nations, the World Health Organization and UNICEF. The views expressed are, however, those of the author.

P-86
ISBN 92-5-100412-9

© FAO 1979

Printed in Italy

HUMAN NUTRITION IN TROPICAL AFRICA

UHURU NA SHIBE KUTOKANA NA CHAKULA BORA
— Let freedom and a satisfied stomach come from good food. *May all the dedicated and talented Africans in medical and other fields make this slogan, in its widest context, a reality in the years ahead.*

ACKNOWLEDGEMENTS

Although the main purpose of this book is to deal with problems of human nutrition specific to Africa, I have benefitted tremendously from several excellent textbooks of nutrition designed for use in all parts of the world. I would particularly mention the books by R.S. Goodhart and M.E. Shills (1973); S. Davidson, R. Passmore, J. Brock and A.S. Truswell (1972); H.C. Trowell and D.B. Jelliffe (1958); and H.C. Trowell, J.N.P. Davies and R.F.A. Dean (1954). All of these are more detailed than the present text, all are worthy of consultation by readers wishing to pursue further certain aspects of nutrition, and I acknowledge that all have been frequently consulted and extensively used in the preparation of this book.

Since this book is likely to be used mainly where scientific library facilities are not available, it was decided not to include a comprehensive list of references. I can therefore only in a general way acknowledge the assistance of the many hundreds of publications including books, pamphlets, and scientific papers that have either been consulted or whose publication has led to the sum total of knowledge that goes to make possible a textbook of nutrition today.

I am grateful for permission to publish in the text a number of photographs from the Tanzania Information Service, which has been most helpful in providing them. Some were taken by Dr J.R.K. Robson. The photographs of Bitot's spots (Figure 39) were provided by Dr D.S. McLaren.

Acknowledgements are also due to the following authors and publishers for the plates indicated: *Tropical nutrition and dietetics*, by L. Nicholls, London, Ballière, Tindall and Cox, photographs on keratomalacia and rickets; Standards for subcutaneous fat in British children by Tanner and Whitehouse, *British Medical Journal*, 17 February 1962, photograph on skinfold calipers; *Diseases of children in the subtropics and tropics* by H.C. Trowell and D.B. Jelliffe, London, Arnold, photograph of nutritional marasmus. Other photographs were supplied by UNICEF and FAO.

I also wish to acknowledge the interest, encouragement and active help of members of the Nutrition Unit and African Regional Office of the World Health Organization; of members of the Nutrition and Rural Institutions and Services Divisions of the Food and Agriculture Organization of the United Nations, both in Rome and in East Africa; and the African Regional and Headquarters Offices of the United Nations Children's Fund.

I am deeply indebted to Dr F.J. Stare, Professor and Chairman of the Department of Nutrition, and Dr D.M. Hegsted, Professor of Nutrition at Harvard University, for a great deal of assistance and advice in the final preparation of the first edition of this book. During the writing of this second edition I constantly obtained guidance and help of all kinds from Dr Lani Stephenson, who is an experienced nutritionist, a collaborator in research in Africa, and also my wife. Her companionship, wisdom and encouragement contributed enormously to the completion of the task. I owe a deep debt of gratitude to her.

MICHAEL C. LATHAM

O.B.E.; B.A., M.B., B.Ch., B.A.O. (Dublin), D.T.M. & H. (London) M.P.H. (Harvard)
Professor of International Nutrition, Cornell University, Ithaca, New York, USA.
Formerly Medical Officer i/c Nutrition Unit, Ministry of Health,
Dar es Salaam, Tanzania
Visiting Professor, University of Nairobi, Kenya
External Examiner, University of Ibadan, Nigeria

NOTE

Vernacular words (in italics) have been used in certain parts of the text in cases where the vernacular (mostly Kiswahili) word is generally known, or is more descriptive, or where there is no exact English equivalent. A glossary of these is given in Appendix 5.

References to dollars ($) are to United States dollars. The monetary unit in Kenya is the shilling (KSh). The value of the shilling in April 1979 was $US 1 = KSh 7.43.

Besides the common abbreviations, symbols and terms, the following have been used in this book:

Nutritional and technical abbreviations

ANP	Applied nutrition programme
BMR	Basal metabolic rate
CSB	Corn/soybean (mixture)
CSM	Corn/soybean/milk (mixture)
DPT	Triple antigen (diptheria, pertussis, tuberculosis vaccine)
DSM	Dried skim milk
ECG	Electrocardiograph
IU	International units
NRC	Nutrition rehabilitation centre
PEM	Protein-energy malnutrition
SCOM	Sugar/casein/oil/milk (mixture)
TMR	Toddler mortality rate

CONTENTS

PREFACE TO THE SECOND EDITION

Fourteen years have passed since this book was first issued. A measure of its impact and usefulness is the fact that it has been necessary to reprint it seven times. This may also be a reflection of the growing interest in human nutrition — and particularly nutrition of the young — being taken by national authorities in tropical Africa.

In view of this sustained demand, the author was called upon to revise, update and expand the manual. He did much of the writing while on sabbatical leave from Cornell University at the University of Nairobi in 1976.

The second edition follows the same format and is aimed at the same audience as the first edition, but in many ways this is a new book. Very intensive revisions have been made, and much new material has been introduced; no chapter has escaped changes and updating. Nutrition is a dynamic subject, and in the years since first publication much new knowledge has been gained; as far as possible this has been incorporated in the new edition. New chapters included are those on food and nutrition policy, government organization for nutrition planning, and nutrition programmes and health strategies. New tables have been added on anthropometric measurements commonly used to assess nutritional status. The tabulated data on recommended dietary intakes and on food composition have been thoroughly revised in the light of current knowledge.

FROM THE PREFACE TO THE FIRST EDITION

More than half the human race is either undernourished or malnourished ... When we consider that in the twentieth century one child out of three is born without any chance of living a normal life, we are forced to conclude that our civilization is mutilating its human resources and reducing its chances of progress ...

It is intolerable that the vast reservoir of knowledge and wealth which exists in the world is hardly being used for improving the lot of the

1

many who are desperately in need of it. Of the several wants of man, food is primary. Hunger and malnutrition can impede the progress of a nation in every other sphere.

These words are from the opening passages of a manifesto (FAO, 1963) issued in Rome by 53 prominent world personalities, many of them Nobel Prize winners. The historic document concludes:

We desire to state with all the emphasis at our command that freedom from hunger is man's first fundamental right. In order to achieve this, we suggest urgent and adequate national and international effort in which the governments and the peoples are associated ... We feel that international action by abolishing hunger will reduce tension and improve human relationships by bringing out the best instead of the worst in man.

A statement produced by distinguished men of many nationalities and races, it has done much to highlight the tremendous importance of nutrition as a problem of people everywhere. It has been said that the history of nutrition is the history of mankind on this planet.

This book was undertaken at the request of international agencies, one of which, FAO, arranged for the special assembly that issued the manifesto quoted above. If this manual can in a modest way help to solve the problems that deeply concerned those men and women, then it has served its purpose.

Despite the international nature of the problems, and although the "have" nations possess a responsibility to assist the "have-not" nations, it is nevertheless vital that the latter countries make every effort themselves. The eventual solutions to these problems must come from within. "God helps those who help themselves", or, as the Koran says, "Man should so use the bounties provided for his sustenance that he should not suffer from hunger".

The nutritional problems, and therefore their solutions, vary from region to region, country to country, area to area. The situation, too, especially in the fast-developing countries, is continually changing. Thus, in much of Africa, although the spread of western ideas has increased the desire for education and for material possessions and has led to vast improvements in many spheres including health, it has done little to reduce the extent of malnutrition and in some instances it has directly created new and serious nutritional problems.

In Africa the problem is not always so much a lack of food as a lack of knowledge about food. For this reason nutrition education in its widest context should be the spearhead of the attack on malnutrition.

This book has been written specifically for the use of health and nutrition workers in Africa, with special reference to the community-health problems of East Africa. Those using it may include assistant medical officers, medical assistants, health inspectors, health nurses, nurses, midwives, nutritionists or similar staff. It might also serve as an introduction to the nutritional problems of the region for doctors and other post-graduate workers entering the field for the first time.

It is assumed that readers have had some scientific education conducted in English, and that they are conversant with general medical terminology. In all the countries of Africa where English is the second language, this is the case for the type of medical worker mentioned above.

Although the most important nutritional work in a community consists of the prevention rather than the cure of nutritional disease, it is still vitally necessary that the basic principles of nutrition be grasped, and also that the clinical aspects of the subject be understood. Without this knowledge, it is impossible to adapt advice and action to suit each area. Improving personal and public health by better nutrition requires ingenuity and knowledge so that sensible practical solutions can be found for each new situation.

The reader must understand, however, that although he or she should know, for example, the names of the main vitamins and the importance of amino acids in protein, it is quite unrealistic and completely unnecessary to use these technical terms when giving nutritional advice to ordinary people who make up the community. This book is designed to teach the health worker how to gauge scientifically what the problems are in a family or a community, in an institution or a district, and to suggest specific ways in which problems can be approached and solved.

The nutritional problems of a community are best tackled cooperatively, by a team approach. Although the book has certain sections and chapters that may be suitable for non-medical members of a team working on various aspects related to nutrition, such as agriculture, community development or education, the book has been written primarily for the health worker. It is for this reason that details are not given of many non-medical solutions to nutritional problems. Although this book may suggest ideas for solving certain problems, it will be necessary for readers who are interested in pursuing further the agricultural, horticultural, educational, or sociological aspects of applied nutrition to consult other works.

When studying human nutrition, it is important to remember that in Africa, in contrast to Europe or America, a far higher percentage, often over half, of the population consists of children. Because children are more vulnerable than most adults to the ravages of poor nutrition, this book stresses the importance of nutrition during childhood. At this period of life, a good, balanced diet will assist optimum development,

3

will allow maximum benefits from education and will help ensure in the next generation a sturdy, healthy society of adults ready to carry the new nations of Africa to their goals.

As President Nyerere said in a broadcast to his nation:

If Tanzania is to give its children the heritage of health as well as freedom, the people must change their attitude toward food. They must learn from each other and from the world about the kinds of foodstuffs which make a man healthy. We have said on many occasions that the three enemies are poverty, ignorance, and disease. By learning about better diet and by using this knowledge, we shall be reducing our ignorance, overcoming many of our diseases, and getting ourselves in a much better position to overcome our poverty. We shall be building up the nation's most important asset — that is, ourselves as human beings.

I. PUBLIC HEALTH ASPECTS OF NUTRITION

1. NUTRITION, INFECTION AND DISEASE

In many developing countries malnutrition is the single most important public-health problem. Yet the ministries of health, and before them the colonial medical departments, have tended to regard nutrition as being of secondary importance.

If an infectious disease were to kill even one quarter of the number of people that kwashiorkor or marasmus kills on average in a year, an urgent control campaign would be mounted. The relative neglect of the morbidity and mortality associated with malnutrition is partly due to its effects being most frequently seen in young children, and because it is not a communicable disease. Furthermore, malnutrition tends to be greatly underreported in disease and mortality statistics. This is because many children recorded as having died of, for example, gastro-enteritis or pneumonia may also have been suffering from malnutrition. Such neglect is shortsighted because undernutrition and malnutrition are serious conditions in themselves and, even when mild or subclinical, may affect the extent and the outcome of other diseases. Economic advancement is to a large measure dependent upon their solution.

A person who is undernourished is much more likely to succumb to an infectious disease than one of good nutritional status. It has been shown that infectious diseases of childhood, such as measles and whooping cough, may precipitate the onset of protein-energy malnutrition. Thus, a seemingly healthy child may develop measles and end up with measles and kwashiorkor. In any attempt, therefore, to improve the nutritional status of children, a parallel attack should be made on the infectious diseases of childhood.

Immunization against whooping cough (pertussis) is a well-established prophylactic procedure. The vaccine is usually combined in a single ampoule with diphtheria and tetanus vaccines; this is known as the DPT vaccine. Inoculations against polio (poliomyelitis) and smallpox are often given

5

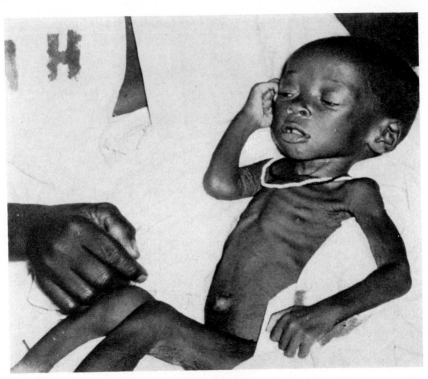

FIGURE 1. Child with marasmus and tuberculosis.

at the same time. Inoculation against measles can also be very effective. However, the vaccine is relatively expensive, has to be kept at all times in a refrigerator and is not yet universally used in Africa. Measles is frequently fatal in young children if the child is poorly nourished; in the child who survives, the disease may lead to loss of weight or may precipitate malnutrition.

Protection of children against these diseases is undoubtedly worthwhile in itself and will also reduce the incidence of protein-energy malnutrition.

Tuberculosis is another important disease in Africa. In infancy this disease is often associated with nutritional marasmus (see Fig. 1). The patient with pulmonary tuberculosis nearly always shows signs of malnutrition. BCG vaccination against tuberculosis is now quite widely used in Africa.

Malaria, another great public-health problem in Africa, tends to be aggravated by malnutrition. Intestinal parasites, which may be extremely common, are also closely linked with malnutrition. It is well established that hookworms, which suck blood, cause a loss of iron and other nutrients.

Roundworms, although large in size and liable to be numerous in the intestine, have not been shown to contribute to malnutrition. Other intestinal parasites play varying roles in malnutrition.

Many infectious diseases, especially those that lead to a rise in temperature (fever), cause an increased loss of nitrogen in the urine. This nitrogen comes from the chemical breakdown of the muscles, and has to be replaced by adequate amounts of protein in the child's food during the period of recovery.

Loss of appetite, known as anorexia, is another factor in the relationship between infection and nutrition. When a child is ill with an infectious disease he often has a poor appetite and therefore a reduced food intake.

More important than any other disease in the aetiology of malnutrition is diarrhoea. This condition may be especially common around the time of weaning and is then sometimes termed "weanling diarrhoea". It is possible that protein-energy malnutrition can be precipitated by an attack of diarrhoea, because diarrhoea seriously interferes with the absorption of food from the gastrointestinal tract in a child who is already poorly nourished. Diarrhoea in an African toddler is frequently treated at home with a bland, mainly carbohydrate diet or by semi-starvation, thus further reducing the food intake.

Antibiotics given for diarrhoea at the dispensary or hospital outpatient department may interfere with the normal intestinal flora and in this way worsen the nutritional state of the child. The old injunction to "starve a fever" is of doubtful validity, and this practice may have serious consequences for the child who is already undernourished. Non-infective diarrhoea may follow a change of diet such as occurs when a child is suddenly taken off the breast and expected to share an often unsuitable family diet. A child fed on breast milk receives a diet with a high nutritive value that is less likely to be contaminated than other foods. The child taken off the breast onto a starchy diet may develop a lowered resistance and is more exposed to gastrointestinal infections.

While diarrhoea can cause malnutrition, kwashiorkor and marasmus are very frequently accompanied by diarrhoea. A grossly deficient diet, especially one deficient in protein, may lead to a reduced secretion of digestive enzymes, particularly from the pancreas. This lack of enzymes may cause non-infective metabolic diarrhoea. Protein-energy malnutrition may therefore be caused by, as well as be a cause of, diarrhoea.

This relationship between diarrhoea and protein-energy malnutrition is stressed because it is desirable that public-health workers consider improving nutrition as a means of lessening the impact of diarrhoeal diseases, and also that medical nutritionists consider using public-health measures to reduce the prevalence of malnutrition.

7

Infections and parasites may be important not only in the aetiology of protein-energy malnutrition and anaemia, as already mentioned, but may also aggravate conditions such as xerophthalmia (due to vitamin A deficiency), an important cause of blindness.

Malnutrition has been clearly shown to lower the body's resistance to infection. A malnourished child has a reduced ability both to form antibodies and to produce increased numbers of white blood cells (leucocytes). These are two very important defence mechanisms. Certain deficiency diseases may impair the integrity of epithelial tissues, notably the skin and mucosae, thus allowing an easy avenue of entry for pathogenic organisms. Vitamin A deficiency is an example of this.

A dramatic illustration of the effect of malnutrition on infection is seen in the high fatality rates of common childhood diseases such as measles. Measles is a severe disease with a case fatality rate of around 15 percent in many African countries, because the young children who develop it have poor nutritional status and low resistance. The death rate from measles in poor countries may be 300 times higher than in the industrialized countries.[1]

It is quite clear that the simultaneous presence of both malnutrition and infection will result in an interaction with more serious consequences for the child than the additive effect of the two working independently. This interaction is known as a synergistic effect. Infections make malnutrition worse, and poor nutrition increases the severity of infectious diseases.

These facts illustrate the importance of a broad, combined attack on public-health problems as part of a campaign to improve nutrition. It is equally important that more attention be paid to nutrition as an integral part of public-health work.

2. AETIOLOGY OF MALNUTRITION

A deficient intake of energy or of a particular nutrient is the cause of most forms of malnutrition. Thus kwashiorkor may be due to a deficient intake of protein and energy, xerophthalmia to inadequate vitamin A or carotene in the diet, and goitre to insufficient iodine. But the fact that we know what nutrient deficiency causes the malnutrition that we see and diagnose does not mean that we understand the often complex un-

---

[1] In the author's experience, working in several African hospitals, it was extremely uncommon for fatalities from measles to occur among children from families of moderate income — such as those of hospital employees or schoolteachers — during a measles epidemic that was causing considerable mortality among the children of poorer families.

8

derlying causes of the disease. Until we understand these, it is difficult to suggest feasible methods for control of malnutrition.

Four particularly important and broad causes of malnutrition in Africa are: a lack of knowledge about food nutrition and health; an insufficient supply of the foods necessary for a balanced diet, due often to lack of production; an uneven distribution of the food that is available; and infectious diseases.

Lack of knowledge

One cannot blame people for their lack of knowledge. Nobody blamed Vasco da Gama when, during the first sea voyage around Africa from Europe to India, 100 out of 180 of his crew died of scurvy. They died because he and they were ignorant of the fact that vitamin C in fresh food prevented scurvy. These people died of scurvy because of lack of knowledge, just as dozens of children are today dying in villages all over Africa because their mothers do not know what foods are necessary to prevent their illness.

Among African and other people, there is a very widespread lack of understanding of the function of food. One of the main aspects of this problem is the general and quite false assumption that "a full belly" is all that is necessary of food to provide health. It is this "full belly" concept, this ignorance, that causes many of the nutritional diseases in these countries. To many people, it is incomprehensible that a person who is never hungry can suffer from a physical disease because of lack of something in the diet.

The author has often had occasion, during his work in Tanzania, to explain to parents of a child suffering from kwashiorkor that the disease is due to a poor diet. The parents have often expressed anguished disbelief that their child could suffer from malnutrition. "This child has never been hungry" they say. "Whenever it cries or needs food we feed it — we give it as much *uji* as it wants and can eat". The parents do not appear to realize that *uji* alone, especially if made only of cassava or maize, is not sufficient to protect a young child from malnutrition, however much it receives.

Another fact that people are often unaware of is the need to feed the young child fairly frequently. Adults and older children may be able to get all their nutritional requirements in two meals a day. But an infant or preschool-age child cannot, especially if the staple food is a bulky, carbohydrate-rich food like plantain, cassava, sweet potatoes or yams, or even a cereal such as maize, millet, rice or wheat. The child does not usually have the appetite or capacity to take in half its daily requirements

9

at one feeding. Therefore, although it may be time-consuming and difficult for mothers, it is important that infants and young children be fed more often than twice a day. Ideally, infants under 1 year of age should be fed six times a day; children 1 to 3 years of age, four to five times a day; and older children, three times a day. How this can be done is discussed in Chapter 8.

Lack of production and supply

The amount of food available for human consumption each year in Africa is unknown. Although it is probable that there is no gross overall shortage in a year of average harvests, in some areas there is undoubtedly a "hungry" season at the end of each agricultural year, before the new harvest is gathered. At this time some people do not get enough to eat.

There have also been widespread famines in certain years (as in the Sahel zone in the mid-1970s), and in parts of East Africa localized famines and food shortages occur quite often. This is true, for example, in the more arid northern parts of Kenya, certain areas of Ethiopia and the Central Region of Tanzania.

There are many reasons why food production in a particular area or by certain families may be low. It can be affected by climatic conditions, the suitability of the soil for certain crops, limited knowledge of agriculture, the availability of seeds, tools, time spent working the land, etc. Sometimes farmers tend to devote too much of their time and land to the cultivation of cash crops and too little to food crops. This may lead to food shortages or poor diets, frequently only partially alleviated by food purchases with the extra money from the sale of the cash crop.

Uneven distribution of food

Food can be unevenly distributed both within the family itself, and within the region as a whole.

Within the family the nutritionally vulnerable members often have lowest priority and therefore little choice of what food is available at any meal. It is a custom in many parts of Africa for the males of the household to eat first. The most tasty portions of the meal are often those that are most nutritious, and little of these are left for the children who come last.

Poor distribution of food in a country as a whole may be the result of a lack of certain foods in some areas (i.e., no cattle in tsetse fly-infested areas, a lack of fruit and vegetables where it is arid, no fish in areas not on

10

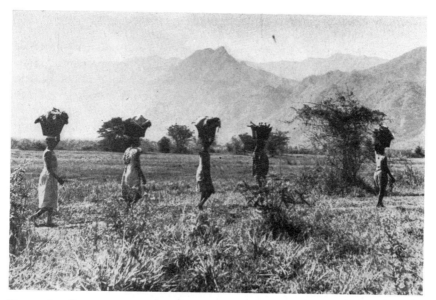

FIGURE 2. Slow transport may limit the distribution of food.

the sea or lakes). These localized shortages of commodities available in the rest of the country are aggravated by poor communications and transport (see Fig. 2) and by lack of storage and preservation facilities.

Uneven distribution in a community may be due to poverty. Foods rich in animal protein and fat are more expensive than predominantly carbohydrate foods. Persons who are not themselves producers of food may not be able to buy nutritious foods simply because they do not have sufficient money. This occurs more commonly among people who are dependent on wages, and frequently in urban areas. A worker on the minimum wage with a lactating wife and three children, for example, usually cannot afford to buy sufficient food to maintain himself and his family in a good nutritional state and at the same time meet the cost of fuel, housing and clothing. The rural employee is in a better position. His wife can still find land on which to grow food, and she can forage for wild leaves and wild fruit. It is clear that in order to have a healthy urban community, one or all of the following must occur: wages must increase in relation to the cost of basic foodstuffs; a meal must be provided at work, or rations supplied; families should be given information on and access to family planning practices in order to allow them to limit their family size to the number they can afford to feed properly; means must be found to allow the urban worker to produce some of his own food, for example, in allotments or backyard gardens.

Infectious diseases

Infectious and parasitic diseases are prevalent in all the countries of Africa. Young children are especially affected. As discussed previously, these contribute notably to malnutrition. Few children with severe protein-energy malnutrition or xerophthalmia do not have a history of a recent or concurrent attack of an infectious or parasitic disease. Similarly, infectious diseases are rendered more serious by malnutrition or undernutrition in the child.

A lack of knowledge about food and nutrition, an insufficient production and supply of food, an uneven distribution of food, and infectious diseases are, as has been stated, among the fundamental causes of malnutrition in Africa. They are related to other factors, including:

— Loss of food through destruction by insects, fungi, rodents, birds, and other animals, such as baboon, wild pig, elephant and porcupine;
— Soil erosion, often resulting from overstocking and indiscriminate burning (see Fig. 3);

FIGURE 3. Soil erosion, often due to overstocking and burning, may render good agricultural land useless.

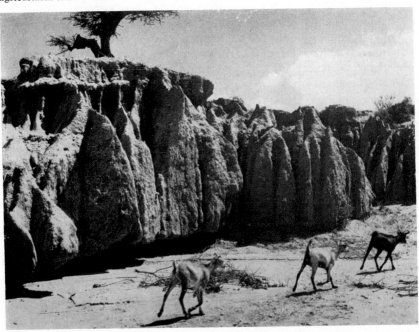

12

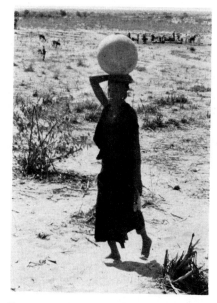

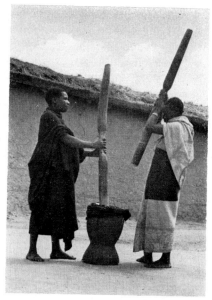

FIGURE 4. Water often has to be collected a long way from the household.

FIGURE 5. Grain preparation is a time-
consuming and arduous procedure.

— Poor farming practices often due to a lack of knowledge, money, time, or equipment;

— Lack of water, which may be of localized, seasonal, or irregular occurrence. Outright failure of the rains may cause famine;

— Lack of time to produce food, prepare it properly and provide special dishes for young children. Among the time-consuming and energy-expending activities of the rural African housewife are the drawing and carrying of water over long distances (see Fig. 4), and the preparation and hand-pounding of cereal grains (see Fig. 5). The provision of adequate water near the house and facilities for lightly milling grain would relieve a woman of a tremendous burden and allow her more time to prepare the foods desirable for young children. Community grouping schemes such as the *ujamaa* villages in Tanzania are a step in the right direction;

— Overpopulation and land shortage, which are serious problems in certain areas of rural Africa;

— Large families raised in households with too little land or income;

— Urbanization and rapid migration to the larger towns resulting in unemployment and low incomes.

It is clear that better agricultural products and methods — such as higher-yielding crop varieties and improved quality of seeds, greater use of fertilizer and insecticides, improved food storage — would make more food available for human consumption per unit of land. However, in many areas of the world the population is increasing at a greater rate than agricultural production. This is a serious problem in much of Asia, where there is frequently not sufficient land to produce the food necessary for the people in a given area. Fortunately, except in a few districts, there is adequate land in East Africa, and therefore the potential to produce all the food necessary for the good health of all the people. Occasionally, however, one finds an inequitable system of land tenure that does not allow optimum use of available agricultural land.

3. NUTRITION, FERTILITY AND FAMILY PLANNING

The world population is expanding at a tremendous rate. Perhaps the major problem in the world is the race between population and food supplies. The world population was around 250 million people 2 000 years ago. After taking 16 centuries to double to 500 million, it then doubled in two and a half centuries to reach 1 000 million in 1850, and doubled again in one century to reach 2 000 million people in 1950. Now the population of the world is doubling every 35 years.

Population pressure is most marked, and is creating major problems, in Asian countries such as Bangladesh, India, Pakistan and Sri Lanka. China has the largest population but its Government has managed in recent years to ensure that its people are adequately fed and has also managed to prevent any large increase in population.

Africa as a whole may not be overpopulated at present, although land pressure is a problem in certain areas. However, the rate of population increase in certain African countries is among the highest in the world. For example, the rate of population increase in Kenya is about 3.5 percent per year; at this rate the population will double in 22 years. The country may well have sufficient land, food-producing capacity and other resources to meet the demands of double or triple the present number of people. But if the goals of development and of an improved quality of life are to be achieved it must be remembered that a doubling of the population in a period of 22 years means that just to maintain the current level of development, there must also be a doubling of the number of schools or school places, of hospitals or hospital beds, of houses and of all services during that same period. While each government must take its own decision concerning a population policy, if the nutritional status of its people is

14

to improve overall, then the availability of food must increase more rapidly than the population.

Family planning, however, is of concern more to the family than to the nation. It is not a question of outsiders trying to limit the total number of children a couple should bear, but rather of giving the couple a means of determining themselves how many children they will have and at what intervals. It becomes a question of the number they want and the spacing between each child.

Family planning is intimately related to health and nutritional status because, for example, large family size, short intervals between children and abrupt termination of breast-feeding are all associated with ill health, including malnutrition, and even increased mortality rates in the mother and family.

Another issue of importance is that it should be a human right for a family, and particularly for women, to choose whether, and when, to have children. This used to be a luxury enjoyed only by those who had the knowledge to practise contraception and the funds to purchase devices. Increasingly, family-planning education is making couples aware of the means of preventing unwanted pregnancies and at the same time programmes are providing contraceptive materials free or at low, highly subsidized prices.

Nutritional status and reproduction

A high number of pregnancies and lactations, especially at short intervals, are likely to deplete the mother of nutrients unless she is receiving an exceptionally good diet. Therefore, women with many children narrowly spaced are likely to have poor nutritional status.

A woman receiving a deficient diet, especially one providing too little total quantity of food and energy, will often give birth to a baby that is smaller than if she were adequately nourished during pregnancy. Since mortality is more likely in underweight babies, poor maternal diets are readily seen to increase the chances of death in the baby. A study in Guatemala showed that supplementing the diets of pregnant women resulted in the mothers producing infants with higher birth weights.

It has also been shown that a short interval between successive children may increase their risk of malnutrition and even of dying, particularly children of birth order five and above. Pregnancies that are too numerous and too narrowly spaced may be harmful both to the mother and child. A mother practising family planning simply to space her children more widely benefits also in nutrition and health. When women are grossly undernourished or starved, as in severe famines, it is usual for them to

15

cease menstruation. This is nature's way of preventing conception in such individuals.

Breast-feeding, fertility and family planning

For many years it was considered to be an old wives' tale that lactation prevented pregnancy. Although it is true that a woman who is still breast-feeding her child may become pregnant, it is now certain that women breast-feeding their babies tend to have a longer period before menstruation begins again, and therefore are less likely to have an early pregnancy than those women who do not breast-feed. Breast-feeding is likely to lengthen birth intervals by an average of 5 to 8 months. In this way prolonged full breast-feeding in developing countries is having a major effect in reducing fertility, in population control, and in child-spacing. It is nature's way of helping to space children. If bottle-feeding were to replace breast-feeding without the availability of contraceptives, it would lead to major increases in the number of children born.

The contraceptive pill, especially if it is a high-oestrogen pill, may reduce the woman's ability to produce breast milk. Therefore care must be taken in advising women soon after birth to take contraceptive pills. In contrast there is a suggestion that the IUD (intra-uterine device) may enhance, or improve, lactation. Some contraceptives may have an effect on nutritional status. Certain of the contraceptive pills are believed to cause anaemia because they affect folate utilization. The IUD may cause increased bleeding, which can lead to iron-deficiency anaemia.

It seems likely that a decrease in infant and child mortality is a prerequisite to the wide acceptance of family planning in those societies in which childhood deaths are common. As malnutrition is one of the leading causes or contributory causes of deaths in children it follows that improved nutrition will expedite the acceptance of family planning. Families need to have confidence that their children will survive before they will risk limiting their family size.

Improved nutrition is part and parcel of a better quality of life. Fewer children in a family means more food, more room and less poverty; these also contribute to an improved quality of life. Wider spacing of children results in improvements in the health and nutritional status of children and their mothers. There is thus a circular effect.

There is much sense in linking, and even in integrating, nutrition and family-planning activities into one programme. Both are related to maternal and child health, and to total family-health care. It may be advantageous for the same health personnel to deal with nutrition, family planning and maternal and child health.

16

4. SOCIAL AND CULTURAL FACTORS IN NUTRITION

It is possible that traditional food practices and taboos constitute an important cause of malnutrition in some areas of Africa. But, in general, cultural food practices are very seldom the main or even an important overriding cause of malnutrition.

All people have their likes and dislikes, and their beliefs about food, yet most are conservative in their food habits. They tend to like what their mothers cooked for them when they were young, and what was served to them at school. If it happened to be baboon flesh, then they will probably never have an aversion to this meat. The foods that people ate without a second thought in childhood are seldom disagreeable to them in later life.

Individuals are further influenced by friends, by what those around them eat, and by what foods are thought to be sophisticated, expensive, or are popularly considered good for health. There is a dislike of being conspicuous or different from others in the same society with regard to foods eaten. Eating habits, however, can be changed as a result of both the influence of other people and sensible adaptation to local circumstances.

Food habits differ most widely in regard to foods of animal origin. Few people have strong feelings about cereals or roots, vegetables or fruits. The foods in question are therefore usually those rich in protein. Because protein is deficient in many African diets, encouragement, not discouragement, should be given to the consumption of any foods of animal origin, irrespective of how bizarre they may seem. The sophisticated, educated man is doing a disservice to his community if after his life in the city, he returns to his village and tells his family and friends that it is disgusting to eat lake flies or locusts, cats or canines, or rodents. Equally, the person who has a liking for some of these unusual protein-rich foods is doing a service to his community if he persuades others to try them.

The child at school is still forming his tastes. If he is introduced to a new food, he will often readily accept it and like it. School meals may usefully serve to introduce new foods to children, and therefore influence food habits. This widening of food experience in childhood is extremely important. The child himself may influence his immediate family and later his own children to eat new, highly nutritious foods.

Good traditional food habits

The traditional diets of most African peoples are good. They usually only need minor changes to allow them to satisfy the nutrient requirements of all members of the family. The problem is not what foods are eaten but rather how much of each food is eaten and how this is distributed within the family.

The habit of eating certain protein-rich foods such as insects, snakes, baboons, mongooses, dogs, cats, unusual seafoods, and snails is definitely beneficial. Another habit that is good nutritionally is the consumption of animal blood. Some tribes puncture the vein of a cow, draw off a calabash of blood, arrest the bleeding, and consume the blood, usually after mixing it with milk. Blood is a rich food and mixed with milk is highly nutritious.

A custom frequently found among African peoples is the drinking of milk sour or curdled, rather than fresh. The souring of milk has little effect on its nutritive value, but the souring process often substantially reduces the number of pathogenic organisms present. In communities where milking is not hygienically performed and where the containers into which the milk goes are likely to be contaminated, it is safer to drink sour rather than fresh milk. Boiled milk, of course, would be safer still.

The traditional use of certain dark green leaves among rural peoples is another beneficial practice and should be encouraged. Such dark green leaves are rich sources of carotene, ascorbic acid, iron and calcium; they also contain useful quantities of protein. Non-cultivated or wild dark green leaves such as amaranth (*mchicha*) and also those from cultivated food crops, such as pumpkin, sweet potato and cassava, are very much richer in vitamins than the pale, leafy European-type vegetables such as cabbage and lettuce. All too often, well-meaning expatriate horticulturists in Africa have tried to get villagers to cultivate lettuce, cabbage, and so on, rather than their traditional vegetables. Many wild fruits are also rich in vitamin C. For example, the pulp within the pod of the frequently consumed baobab has a high vitamin C content.

Traditional methods of grain preparation produce a more nutritious product than does elaborate machine milling.

Some communities sprout legume seeds prior to cooking, which enhances their nutritive value. This also applies to the soaking of whole grain cereals, which is done before making many local beers (*pombe*) and some non-alcoholic beverages (e.g., *togwa*). All these usually have a high vitamin B content.

Finally, it cannot be stressed too strongly that for most African mothers the traditional and natural method of infant feeding from the breast is much superior to bottle-feeding (see p. 43).

Poor food habits and beliefs

There are a number of food habits and practices that are poor from a nutritional point of view. Some are merely traditional views about food

18

that are liable to change under the influence of neighbouring peoples, travel, education, etc. Other food practices are governed by definite taboos. A taboo may have to be followed by a whole tribe, by part of a tribe, or by certain groups within the tribe. Tribes may be divided into subtribes and clans, lineages and families, any of which may have different food taboos.

Cutting across this and within the tribe or clan, different food customs may be practised only by women or children, or by pregnant women, or by female children. In certain tribes traditional food customs are practised by a particular age group and in other instances a taboo may be linked with an occupation such as hunting. At other times or in other individuals a taboo may be imposed because of some particular event such as an illness or an initiation ceremony.

Although these matters border on the realm of anthropology, it is important for a change agent to be familiar with all the food habits of people in order to be able to improve their nutritional status through nutrition education or other means. A whole book could be written about regional food habits and the taboos of any country. It is evident that anthropology and sociology are important to the nutrition worker who is either investigating or trying to improve the nutritional status of any community.

Some customs and taboos have known origins, and many are often logical, though the original reason for the logic may have disappeared. The custom may become part of the religion of the people involved. For example, the Jewish taboo against pork was probably introduced to get rid of the prevalent pork tapeworm, which was thought to be sapping the strength of the Jewish people. Even 2 000 years later, though now it is possible to eat pork safely, Jews still do not eat pork. African Muslims share this view about pork.

Many taboos in Africa, as elsewhere, unfortunately relate to protein-rich animal foods, and to those groups of the community most in need of protein. A common taboo against the consumption of eggs is rapidly disappearing. This taboo usually applies to females, who are said to become sterile if they eat eggs. The psychological connection between human fertility and the egg is obvious. In other places the custom relates to children, who may have been forbidden to eat eggs in order to discourage them from stealing the eggs of sitting hens, thus endangering the survival of poultry. Elsewhere, a whole tribe may not eat eggs, solely because of a revulsion against them.

Other customs, again often affecting women and children, concern fish. These customs may amount to a full taboo, though people not used to fish often dislike it merely because of its "distasteful" smell or "snake-like" appearance. Other food beliefs concern goat's milk and goat's meat.

19

Some of these seem illogical and their origin is obscure. For example, in some tribes it is said that a child who drinks goat's milk will grow to look like a goat.

In the past some communities had such a wide range of taboos for the pregnant woman that it was practically impossible for her to get a balanced diet. A section of the Bahaya people living near Lake Victoria used to forbid the consumption by pregnant women of meat, fish, milk, and eggs.

Many of the bad food habits and taboos that existed in Africa a quarter of a century ago have already disappeared or are rapidly doing so, as a result of education, mixing of tribal groups, greater travel, and also as a result of the sense of nationhood replacing tribalism in the newly independent states. It is not advisable for outsiders to try to alter ancient food habits without looking very closely into their origins. It is better for influential local people to try to change nutritionally bad habits. A speech by the president or a cabinet minister, the sight of a respected leader of the tribe eating some "forbidden" food and coming to no harm, the return to the village of educated and enlightened local people will all prove much more effective than the preaching or goading of an outsider.

Changing food habits

In some parts of Africa the staple foods are changing. For example, maize, cassava and potatoes, now grown in large amounts in Africa, originated outside the continent. Since none of these foods were being eaten in Africa a few hundred years ago, it is clear that the food habits of millions have indeed changed. Vast numbers of people in Africa have abandoned yams and millet for maize and cassava, just as many in Europe abandoned oats, barley, and rye for wheat and potatoes. Food habits are still changing rapidly. The difficulty, of course, lies in trying to guide and foster desirable changes and to slow down undesirable ones.

It is difficult to say what stimulates and influences changes. The rapid increase in bread consumption in many African countries is understandable. It is at least in part a labour-saving phenomenon because bread is one of the first "convenience" foods to have become available: the person going to work can have some slices of bread before leaving home, instead of the traditional porridge (*ugali*), which is unpleasant cold, and to prepare fresh and hot requires someone to be up at the cooking stoves well before daybreak. Bread can be carried in the pocket and eaten during a break in the working day, or on safari.

Some tribes have a predilection for one staple food and have no desire to change, as is the case with many banana-eating tribes. But even where the staple food remains unaltered, the form in which it is preferred may change (the rapid spread in popularity of milled white rice in Asia and its disastrous consequences are discussed later). Similarly in eastern and southern Africa, there is a growing demand for very white, fine maize-meal, which is nutritionally inferior to the coarser, darker product.

This desire for a white product is not restricted to Africa or Asia, but is also prevalent in western societies; for example, there was a public outcry in the United Kingdom against the introduction of the non-white loaf of bread during the Second World War. The Russian "black" bread is also rapidly losing favour and being replaced by white bread. Only in the higher-income groups or among food faddists is it becoming sophisticated to swing the pendulum back in favour of brown bread and whole-grain cereal foods.

Harmful new habits

Many changes in food habits that have been introduced or encouraged in Africa by western so-called civilization have been harmful. For example, the change from lightly milled to highly milled cereals is becoming a serious problem in Africa. While it would be unrealistic to suggest that a serious attempt should be made to stop this trend, its effects on the health of the community could be minimized by, for example, introducing legislation to enforce vitamin and mineral enrichment of the deficient cereal products.

Although much has been written about the harmful effects of the spread of bottle-feeding, much less attention has been given to the question of other "baby foods" marketed in Africa. Many of these are convenient to use but very few are superior nutritionally to locally available foods already being used for infant feeding. None of them contain nutrients not present in the recipes given in Part VI, which involve cheap and easily available ingredients.

As with bottle-feeding, no harm is done to the young child of an affluent family using these manufactured products. But for most families in Africa they are a total waste of money and should not be purchased by mothers who already have too little to spend on food. Nearly all these manufactured foods are expensive ways of buying the nutrients they are advertised to contain.

Another particularly misleading type of advertising relates to the "glucose" products said to provide "instant energy". Energy is present in large amounts in nearly all the cheapest foods. Similarly the drinks advertised as being "rich in vitamin C" are usually unnecessary since African children seldom suffer from vitamin C deficiency. They can

21

just as well obtain their vitamin C from fruits such as guavas, mangoes and citrus, or from a range of vegetables.

The so-called protein-rich weaning foods are also much advertised. These are nutritionally good products but their cost is much higher than protein-rich foods such as beans, groundnuts or even dried fish, meat, eggs or milk available in the market. It probably costs more to provide 100 grams of protein from these commercially advertised products than, for example, from beans bought in the local market. The essential question is what is the best that a mother could do to improve her child's diet if she had a little extra to spend. The answer would seldom be a manufactured baby food.

Another, quite different, problem is the tendency of many wage earners to spend almost the whole of their wage within a few days of receiving it. The result is often that the nutritive value of the family diet is much better just after pay day than later in the month. Wages in East Africa are usually paid monthly, and there seems little doubt that, should it prove possible to change prevailing practices to the payment of weekly wages this would tend to improve the diet of the wage earner and his family.

Influencing change for the better

What can health workers or nutritionists in a community do about food habits, old and new?

They can:

- Persuade people to maintain and preserve the many excellent existing food habits that are nutritionally valuable;
- Set good examples in their own households by adopting good food habits and not following food taboos;
- Influence respected local leaders to state publicly that they themselves have dropped food taboos, and arrange for them, when occasion arises, to eat "forbidden" foods in public;
- Persuade people not to abandon good food habits under the influence of "sophisticates" back from the city who may try to discourage rural dwellers from eating such nutritional foods as locusts or lake flies, or those non-Africans and others who try to encourage the consumption and production of European-type vegetables in place of better traditional ones;
- Explain the disadvantages of highly refined cereal flours, if the latter are being preferred, in their area, and advocate the consumption of a range of cereals in the local diet;

- Issue information material to help stop the spread of bottle-feeding and the unnecessary purchase of expensive baby foods;
- Strive, through civil service or local authority organizations, for the introduction of the payment of weekly wages instead of monthly wages to employees. Influence labour and trade union leaders to do the same;
- Take steps to introduce good feeding practices in the local schools.

5. ASSESSMENT OF NUTRITIONAL STATUS

Nutritional problems are complex in their aetiology and the types of information that can be useful in the assessment of nutritional status are numerous and diverse. They are discussed in detail in Jelliffe (1966) and include:

1. Clinical examination data;
2. Anthropometric data;
3. Laboratory tests of nutritional status;
4. Dietary surveys;
5. Vital statistics;
6. Additional health statistics and medical information;
7. Agricultural data relevant to food production and food balance sheets;
8. Economic data related to puchasing power, food prices, food distribution, etc.;
9. Socio-cultural data including food consumption patterns, and food practices and beliefs;
10. Food science information such as the nutrient content of foods, the biological value of diets, the effects on nutrients of common food-processing practices, and the presence of toxic or harmful factors such as aflatoxins and goitrogens.

Only the first five are discussed here since a nutrition survey comprehensive enough to collect all these types of information would very seldom be undertaken.

Large and expensive surveys in which a wide variety of nutrition-related data are collected are seldom justified, and should never be done unless there is a reasonable assurance that the data will be used for an action programme, and that adequate resources and funds are available. In many countries expensive surveys have been carried out and little action has followed. It has been suggested that ten times the amount spent on a survey should be available for programmes aimed at overcoming the deficiencies it identifies.

It is therefore important that the information collected be kept to the minimum required to assess the situation, and that surveys be simplified as much as possible.

The information used for the assessment of the nutritional status of a community can also be used for evaluation of programmes, and for nutritional surveillance (see p. 35).

Clinical examinations

Clinical examinations are often given low priority as a means of assessing the nutritional status of a community. Moreover, most countries in Africa suffer from a lack of vital statistics, accurate figures of agricultural production, and laboratories where biochemical tests can be performed; records of local food habits and practices are difficult to obtain. Under these conditions clinical and anthropometric examinations form the simplest, most practical and without doubt the soundest means of ascertaining the nutritional status of any particular group of individuals.

The nutritional status of a community is the sum of the statuses of the individuals who form that community. However, in any survey only a representative group of persons need be examined. To give a true picture, these should normally be chosen completely at random, not taken from any particular age group, sex or religion, area within the community, or social class. Stratified sampling is valid under certain circumstances. For example, if a survey is being carried out to determine the importance and prevalence of protein-energy malnutrition among the young in a given area, then it would be sound practice to restrict examinations to children up to 5 years of age. If the exact date of birth of the child is unknown then the age should be estimated using local historical, agricultural or social events as time indices.

The clinical nutrition examination should be carried out by a person with medical training. Although it may be possible to train non-medical personnel to recognize such conditions as angular stomatitis, mottled teeth, and even oedema, it is, nevertheless, unwise to have people performing an examination to collect statistical clinical data without a fairly wide knowledge of medicine. It is not recommended that persons without medical training should carry out clinical nutrition examinations. It is desirable, for example, that a person looking for the dermatoses of kwashiorkor or the skin changes of pellagra should also be familiar with the appearance of scabies and eczema. However, non-medical persons can

24

be entrusted to collect anthropometric data (physical measurements).

In order to avoid overlooking important details, the clinical examination should be systematic, with the examiner looking for specific signs. The presence or absence of these signs should be recorded on a standardized form. A modified sample of a form that has been found useful in practice in East Africa over the past few years is given on page 26.

Using this form, examinations should start at the head (i.e., hair, eyes, mouth), move down the body, and end at the feet. Central nervous system (CNS) signs may in some instances be omitted, because they are relatively rare in Africa and the tests may be difficult and time-consuming to perform.

Anthropometric data

Anthropometric data can be collected by medical or non-medical personnel. In the former case, they can be included as part of the clinical nutritional examination. However, it is often simpler and faster if a reliable person other than the medical examiner records the height and weight during a survey.

Weight. The weight of a person is the most important single anthropometric measurement that can be taken. In children its interpretation is dependent on knowing the age of the child with some degree of accuracy.

Weight should be recorded with the subject nude or wearing the minimum of clothing (shorts only for males, light dress for females). Footwear should be removed. The weight of irremovable metal bangles, which are commonly worn in certain parts of Africa, must be taken into account.

Spring scales are less reliable than balance scales. In many parts of Africa, the latter type of scale has been supplied by the United Nations Children's Fund (UNICEF) to clinics and health centres. At boarding schools, a good scale is often available in the kitchen, where it is used for weighing sacks of food. Similarly, in a village, the local market master or the owner of a small shop will usually have a produce scale that can be borrowed. Special baby-weighing scales are necessary for accurate weight measurement of children under 2 years of age.

Height. This is also a very important measurement in the assessment of nutritional status. Like weight, its interpretation in children is dependent on knowing the age of the child.

Height should be measured with the subject barefoot. Though many different types of equipment are available, height can be fairly ac-

Clinical nutrition examination

(For use of medical personnel)

Name ....   Date . . . .
Sex ....   Age ....
Pregnant? ....   Lactating? ....
Height ....   Weight ....
Haemoglobin ....   Upper arm circumference ....
Haematocrit ....   Triceps skin thickness ....

Hair

1. Lack of lustre? ....
2. Dyspigmentation (colour change)?
3. Texture change (thinness or sparseness)? ....
4. Easily pluckable? ....

Face

1. Moonface? ....
2. Pallor? ....

Eyes

1. Xerosis conjunctivae or xerophthalmia? ....
2. Keratomalacia? ....
3. Conjunctival thickening or wrinkling? ....
4. Bitot's spots? ....
5. Conjunctival injection or vascularization? ....
6. Corneal scars? ....

Mouth

1. Angular stomatitis? ....
2. Cheilosis of lips? ....
3. Angular scars? ....
4. Gums spongy or bleeding? .....
5. Mottled teeth? ....
6. No. teeth decayed (D) ....
7. No. teeth missing (M) ....
8. No. teeth filled (F) ....
9. Total DMF teeth ....

Glands

Thyroid
  Goitre
    Grade 0 1 2 3 ....
Parotid enlarged? ....

Skin

1. Xerosis (dry scaly)? ....
2. Follicular hyperkeratosis? ....
3. Mosaic (crazy pavement)? ....
4. Pellagrous dermatosis? ....
5. Skin haemorrhages (petechiae or ecchymoses)? ....
6. Flaky paint dermatosis? ....
7. Scrotal or vulval dermatosis? ......
8. Oedema? ....
9. Ulcers? ....

Muscles

1. Wasting? ....

Skeleton

1. Epiphyseal enlargement? ....
2. Beading of ribs (rickety rosary)? ....
3. Skeletal deformities? ....
4. Subperiosteal haematomas? ....

Central nervous system (CNS)

1. Psychomotor change (apathy, misery, etc.)? ....
2. Sensory loss? ....
3. Calf tenderness? ....
4. Loss of ankle or knee jerks? ......
5. Motor weakness? ....

Internal system

1. Hepatomegaly? ....
2. Splenomegaly? ....

Remarks (include other abnormalities)
....
....
....

curately measured with a tape measure or even a ruler. The following method may be used:

Locate a vertical wall rising from a truly horizontal floor. Make a horizontal pencil line about 2 cm in length at a height of 1 m from the floor (60 cm for children). Then, using sticking plaster, sticky tape, or a drawing pin, secure the bottom of a 1-m length of tape measure to correspond with the line. Similarly fasten the top, which will now be 2 m from the floor. Persons being measured stand against the wall facing outward (see Fig. 6). The height of the individual is ascertained using a block of wood having a true right angle. A rectangular cubed block with the dimensions 30 × 10 × 20 cm is adequate, though a triangular block 30 × 10 × 20 cm in size, as shown in Figure 6, is easier to handle.

The measurement of the height of young children presents more difficulty. A suitable piece of apparatus consists of a flat board of dimensions 120 × 40 × 2 cm with a 30-cm-high headboard fixed at right angles to

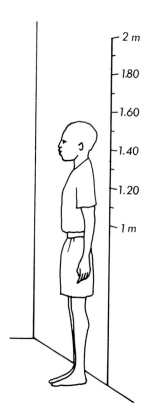

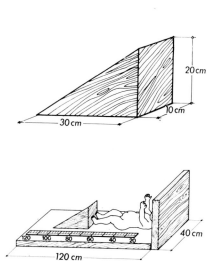

FIGURE 6. *Left:* Measuring height on level floor against a vertical wall. *Above:* Triangular block used in measuring height. *Below:* Measuring height or length of infants.

one end. The triangle used for height measurements can be used as a sliding foot-piece. A metal tape measure is nailed to the board for readings in centimetres.

A less satisfactory alternative is to push a flat wooden bench, available in most dispensaries and schools, up against a wall in the corner of the room and measure it off in centimetres starting about 50 cm from the wall and going up to 150 cm. The triangle is again used as a foot-piece.

When measuring the height of infants and toddlers, the child must lie flat and be straightened out to full length (see Fig. 6).

Types of height and weight measurement

Series readings. A series of readings of weight and/or height of an individual taken at, for example, monthly intervals gives valuable information. In an adult, weight loss indicates that energy intake is below energy output. Gain in weight indicates a more than sufficient energy supply. In adults a series of weight readings might be used, for example, during a famine to ascertain whether relief measures are adequate, or in a normal year to see if weight drop occurs during the "hungry season".

In children a series of monthly height and weight readings gives an extremely valuable record of a child's progress and nutritional status. It is well worth keeping a record of the measurement of heights and weights of children taken in schools, dispensaries, and even community centres. The measurements can be carried out by either medical or non-medical personnel. When done as a series of readings, figures for weight even without those of height are useful.

If single readings of weight or height are available, they can be compared with some standard weight or height. The individual child's actual weight or height can then be expressed as a percentage of that expected for his age. For example, a child of 13 months might be expected to weigh 10 kg. If at that age it weighed only 8 kg it would be 80 percent of the expected weight for its age. Standard tables for weight, height and certain other anthropometric measurements are given in Appendix 2.

Weight for height. When weight and height have both been measured, it is possible to determine how near the child is to the standard of weight for his height. Even if the age of the child is not known it is possible to make some assessment of his nutritional status by determining what percentage his weight is of that expected for his height or length. This figure gives a relative measure of how thin the child is. For example, a child 75 cm in height should, if healthy, weigh about 10 kg (see Table 3 in Appendix 2). One weighing 7 kg would be only 70 percent of the ex-

28

pected weight for his height, and would be classified as a thin child showing evidence of malnutrition. However, such evidence should be treated with caution — in places where there is a great amount of chronic malnutrition, weight-for-height data may be deceptive as weight and height for age may both be reduced while weight/height ratios remain normal.

Mid upper-arm circumference (UAC). The measurement of the circumference of the left upper arm midway between the acromion process of the shoulder and the olecranon process of the elbow is being increasingly used as an index of nutritional status. Fibreglass tape measures that do not stretch should be used. Although this method does not provide as reliable information concerning nutritional status as do weight and height, it has the advantage of being inexpensive and usable where no weighing-scale is available. Furthermore, between about 8 months and 5 years of age the standard arm circumference increases very little. An arm circumference of above 13.5 cm can be considered normal for children from 1 to 5 years of age, one between 12.0 and 13.5 cm as indicating moderate malnutrition and one below 12.0 cm more serious malnutrition. The UAC measurement may be especially suitable for use by persons with a minimum of training, or for gross assessment of nutritional status in famine areas.

Head circumference. This measurement can be made using the same tape measure as for the arm circumference. The tape is placed horizontally around the head at a level just above the eyebrows, the ears and the most prominent bulge at the back of the head. Head circumference is related to brain size, but brain size is not necessarily related to intelligence.

Chest circumference. This is measured horizontally at the nipple line. Up to 6 months of age the head circumference is usually larger than the chest circumference. Children over 12 months of age having a larger head than chest circumference are abnormal. This is evidence of poor growth of the chest.

Skinfold thickness. The skinfold thickness can only be measured if a pair of skinfold calipers is available (see Fig. 7). This instrument is designed to measure the thickness of the skin and subcutaneous fat, using constant pressure applied over a known area. The two commonest sites used are over the triceps and in the subscapular region. The instrument provides a measurement of considerable value in assessing the amount of fat, and therefore the reserve of energy, in the body. Unfortunately there are not many African hospitals, let alone health centres and dispensaries, where this instrument is available. This could easily be rectified, since the instrument is not expensive.

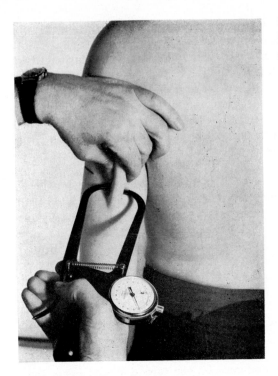

FIGURE 7. The skinfold caliper is used to measure the thickness of the triceps skinfold.

Laboratory tests

There are many laboratory tests of great value in determining nutritional status, but few of these can at present be performed other than in large hospitals. Only those tests that are more widely available are discussed here.

Haemoglobin. An accurate assessment of haemoglobin level is by far the most important laboratory information that can be obtained in any nutrition survey. Accurate haemoglobinometers are all too frequently not available in many district hospitals, health centres and dispensaries. The clinical nutritionist should always have one among his equipment.

The Tallquist or "blotting paper" method of measuring haemoglobin level is inaccurate and of little value in nutritional assessment. In fact a clinical assessment based on degree of pallor of the tongue, conjunctiva and nail bed, and expressed as normal, near normal, mildly anaemic, clearly anaemic, and severely anaemic gives results which are as good and which are less pretentious than the so-called percentage figure of the Tallquist scale.

30

Haematocrit or packed cell volume (PCV). The determination of this is also important in the diagnosis of anaemia. A capillary tube is filled with blood — either venous or finger-prick capillary blood. This is spun in a standardized electric centrifuge, which separates the red cells from the plasma. The haematocrit or PCV indicates the percentage of the blood volume composed of cells.

Red cell counts and blood films. The former are not easy to do and add little information to the above tests. However, it is easy to prepare a thin blood film on a glass slide. Such a slide is useful, since it enables the size and uniformity of the red blood cells to be seen, and may facilitate the diagnosis of malaria and the haemoglobinopathies that may also cause anaemia.

Serum protein. Determination of the total serum protein, and of the serum albumin and globulin levels, can only be undertaken in a well-equipped laboratory. These data give useful information in cases of kwashiorkor, but have not been found to be helpful in the diagnosis of mild or moderate protein-energy malnutrition. The same is true of two other tests — the amino-acid ratio and the hydroxyproline-creatinine index. Neither of these is suitable for the district hospital, health centre or dispensary.

Examination of stools, urine, and blood for parasites. If laboratory tests are being performed during a nutritional survey, the next most important tests after haemoglobin estimation are strictly non-nutritional tests. Nevertheless, as stated earlier, there is little doubt that parasitic infestation and malnutrition are closely linked. The medical nutritionist must examine the individual and the community from all aspects relating to public health. Laboratory examination should therefore be made of stools for the ova of hookworm, roundworm, *Schistosoma mansoni* and other parasites, of urine for albumin, casts, and *S. haematobium*, and of blood for malaria parasites. These tests are all easily performed in most dispensaries. They require only a microscope, a hand centrifuge, some laboratory glassware, and a few simple reagents. Precautions should be taken regarding collection and disposal of specimens. Quantitative tests to assess parasite load should be performed if possible.

During a nutritional survey it may be preferable to do these examinations on a separate day, or during the afternoon following clinical examinations in the morning. In a large community it is advantageous to restrict these examinations to one particular group, such as all the children at the local school. This will give a reasonable picture of the prevalence of diseases such as malaria and ankylostomiasis in the community. It is easier and more hygienic (especially with regard to stool examinations) to deal with a simple group than to collect specimens from people scattered over wide areas who have assembled in large numbers at a centre for clinical examination.

Dietary surveys

It takes much longer to assess accurately the dietary intake of a community than it does to get a picture of their nutritional status by clinical or anthropometric examination. There are two main types of dietary survey. One relies on direct observation, a sample of the population having their food measured and weighed over a given period of time. The other relies on inquiry, with a larger group of people being questioned about their diet. The former method has the disadvantage of being very time-consuming and the latter of depending on the memory, integrity and intelligence of the subjects being questioned. Neither method takes account of past consumption or of uncertainties of food composition. Such definitive methods are rarely justified or practicable; it is often better to use the cruder, simpler methods. These will usually provide data that reveal the causes of malnutrition and that suggest corrective measures.

The different dietary surveys performed will often clearly indicate what is wrong with a diet but they should not be used as a diagnostic method. Conclusions should be drawn only after critically looking at possible sources and margins of error in the method being used.

The difficulties of carrying out a dietary survey using observation methods where food is weighed and measured are discussed below.

Observation. The only way to assess the diet accurately is to weigh and measure all the food that individuals eat over a representative period of time. A survey team goes in groups to households and weighs and measures all food that is prepared, cooked and eaten, as well as that which is wasted or discarded. This procedure should be followed in each household for 3-10 days, and, if possible, repeated at different seasons of the year. Weighing and measuring should be accompanied by inquiry, so as to avoid collecting data on the one day in the month, for instance, when a cow is slaughtered and eaten.

If possible the proportion of the total quantity of food prepared that is eaten by each individual should be weighed. This is difficult in much of Africa, where people often feed from one large communal dish or pot. Having ascertained what each person eats on an average day, it is necessary to calculate the amount of each nutrient eaten by each subject or each family, using quantitative tables of dietary constituents. Dietary surveys in Africa may reveal constituents of the diet that have not previously been analysed. These should be analysed in a laboratory, even if food specimens have to be sent a long distance, or out of the country.

A dietary survey of this kind requires a survey team of at least two persons that can cover two to four families at one time, and perhaps 20 families in a month. It is essential to obtain truly representative households to serve as samples, and to cover a small, statistically acceptable sample of the population properly, rather than to try to cover more families in a less thorough manner.

Inquiry or recall. Direct inquiry cannot give very accurate information on amounts of energy or nutrients consumed. But it can give an indication of the frequency of meals, the methods of food preparation and cooking, as well as providing details of the foods commonly consumed. Only a rough estimate can be made of the amount of each food eaten. Detailed questioning may also give some information about less frequently consumed food.

In Africa it is more usual for a survey worker to go to a household, ask the wife questions about the diet and record the answers on a form. This kind of inquiry depends heavily on the memory of those giving information, and also on their attitude toward the person inquiring. False answers are often given unconsciously. Equally, the subject may have some concealed reason for misleading the inquirer. For example, if the subjects believe that the inquiries are being made to ascertain whether famine-relief food should be issued or increased, then quite naturally they will indicate that they are eating a small quantity and variety of food. If, however, they believe that the questioner is attempting to assess their standard of living or their degree of development, local pride may influence them to indicate that they eat a greater quantity and larger variety of food than is actually the case.

The commonest method is to ask the person to recall what was consumed during the previous 24-hour period. It is useful to have available local measures (bowls, cups, spoons) so that the respondent can indicate the approximate amount eaten.

Another survey method used is to have literate people fill in a questionnaire. For example, schoolchildren are given a questionnaire to complete each morning for a week. They are asked to record what they ate during the last 24 hours. The process should be repeated at different seasons of the year. Such an inquiry gives no indication of quantities consumed. It may, however, provide useful information about meal patterns, the staple foods of each household, the frequency of consumption of meat, fish, eggs, fruit or vegetables, seasonal variations in diets, etc. Food-frequency surveys of this kind can be performed on other groups of people. These provide qualitative, not quantitative, information.

Combined observation and inquiry. A combination method is for the observers to go to previously selected households and to ask the wife to show what food she intends to cook for the family that day. This is then accurately weighed, and the number, sex and age of the people in the household are recorded. The worker then moves on to the next household. Clearly very much more ground can be covered per day using this method than with a full-scale dietary survey as described above.

However, the wife may have no idea of how much food she is going to use that day, or she may exaggerate the amount. This type of survey takes no account of food loss or wastage and gives no indication of what each individual member of the family consumes. The medical nutritionist is often very keen to know what the toddler or the pregnant woman is actually eating, and not what the whole family gets.

One survey using this method, carried out in East Africa under the direction of statisticians, reported that the people surveyed consumed over 5 000 Calories per head per day. Malnutrition and undernutrition were known to exist in this area, and the likely intake of those questioned was 2 200 Calories. Clearly the average householder in this survey area had tried to impress the observer with how well he lived.

Vital statistics

Vital statistics are those related to births and deaths in the community. Complete and accurate vital statistics are not maintained in African countries, nor are they likely to be in the near future. However, vital statistics are so important as an index of nutritional status and for other public-health reasons that they serve a useful purpose even if collected in small areas only.

In industrialized countries, the infant mortality rate (death during the first year of life) gives a good indication of the state of nutrition and the health of the community. The neonatal mortality rate (death during the first month of life) and stillbirth rates are also useful.

In Africa, figures for the toddler mortality rate (TMR — deaths between the first and fifth birthdays) would be far more useful than the other rates to the nutritionist. TMR values often give a good indication of the prevalence of protein-energy malnutrition, although they do not necessarily illustrate the nutritional status of the whole community.

A high TMR due to protein-energy malnutrition may occur in a community where other groups are reasonably nourished and vice versa.

For example, inhabitants of one lakeside community may stop breast-feeding abruptly at around the first birthday. They may regard fish as an unsuitable food for infants, and feed them on little else than porridge made from cassava flour. A high TMR from protein-energy malnutrition would be expected. Yet the nutrition of the older inhabitants of the community, who may eat cassava, fish, groundnuts, and green leaves, might be satisfactory. Another community in, say, arid cattle-country may continue breast-feeding into the second year, gradually weaning the toddler onto a millet porridge mixed with sour milk. The TMR from protein-energy malnutrition would be low, yet the people as a whole might be malnourished due to lack of energy, protein, and vitamins A and C.

The TMR often provides a clear indication of the comparative state of development of a country. For example, in Scandinavia, the USSR, North America and the United Kingdom, the TMR is about 1 per 1 000, while in much of Asia and Africa it is at least 40 times as much. The infant mortality rate is around 10 per 1 000 in Sweden and that in most African countries ranges from 35 to 180 per 1 000.

Although it is normally impossible for an individual worker or a survey team to collect accurate vital statistics, some information of value regarding birth rate and death rate is usually available. For example, during a survey, one can easily ask all married women of child-bearing age two simple questions:

— To how many live children have you given birth?
— How many are still alive today?

From these figures a percentage of children that have died, and also some indication of the fertility rate, can be obtained. Careful questioning might also elicit the approximate ages of the living children and a rough estimate of the age at which the others died. Questioning as to the cause of death rarely produces information of any real value.

All information gained in this way should be cross-checked with a village leader or, in a Christian community, with the local priest or pastor. In Christian communities, baptismal records can be useful in determining the age of children, and burial records can provide death dates.

It must be emphasized that information gathered this way only provides rough estimates of the true figures, but these are nevertheless useful and will have to suffice until such time as proper vital statistics are maintained.

Nutritional surveillance

The term "nutritional surveillance" is used to describe a system of continuous monitoring of certain factors that relate to, or affect, the nutritional status in a community or area; the system should indicate when a nutrition intervention is needed. As yet, no country has an adequate or complete system of nutritional surveillance. However, it should be possible to design surveillance systems that are both simple and yet sensitive enough to detect any change in nutritional status for the worse or better. This could provide an alert before starvation occurred in high-risk famine areas. Ethiopia, India and Mexico have recently adopted some form of nutritional surveillance to assess the nutritional situation at any time in given areas of the country.

Such systems need to be efficiently run because the data collected have to be transmitted rapidly to a centre for analysis; the results are then made available to government authorities for further action.

Example. A country that has had famines in two remote regions decides to establish a surveillance system confined to those high-risk areas. In each region one village in ten is selected at random. Data of three kinds are selected as indicators of famine: the percentage of children between 1 and 5 years of age with an arm circumference below 13 cm; the price of cereal grains and beans in village shops; the weekly rainfall in each village. The medical staff at the dispensary or health centre nearest each village are made responsible for measuring the arm circumference of 100 children from randomly selected households each fortnight; the agricultural extension worker in the area monitors food prices; and the headmaster of each village primary school is provided with a rain gauge to report on rainfall. Every second Saturday the health staff and the agricultural extension officer meet the headmaster at the school, who records the information on a prepared form for immediate mailing to the head office responsible for nutritional surveillance. This office decides on possible interventions on the basis of known relationships between these indicators.

Only three examples of indicators are given here but information on weather, health, food production, pests and many other topics could also give additional useful information.

Some countries in Africa are planning national nutritional surveillance systems. They need to select appropriate indicators, to design a rapid method of data reporting, and to plan a means of response to the findings reported.

6. NUTRITION DURING PREGNANCY

The nutritional needs of a woman during pregnancy (and lactation) are greater than at other times in her life. The reason for this is obvious: a pregnant woman is building up in her own body the tissues and organs

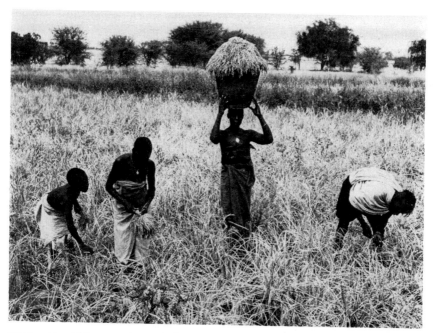

FIGURE 8. African women remain active during pregnancy.

of a new human being. Apart from oxygen, the various elements required are normally provided in the food she eats. This point is stressed in Chapter 2, and is also highlighted in Table 1 of Appendix 1.

A child born to a mother deficient in vitamin A is more likely to develop xerophthalmia or other signs of vitamin A deficiency than one whose mother is on a diet adequate in vitamin A. Similarly, since the infant receives a store of iron from the mother, if she is deficient that store is liable to be smaller. In the case of many other nutrients, however, the child is truly parasitic and takes all the nutrients it requires irrespective of whether the mother is deficient or not. Calcium is one such nutrient, but this does not mean that extra calcium is not desirable during pregnancy. If the mother is not given calcium, she will lose it from her own body to the benefit of the foetus.

Women gain weight during pregnancy, and a heavier person needs more energy to perform the same amount of physical work as a lighter person. In many countries women during pregnancy live an easy life, rest frequently or do not work, thus reducing their energy needs. However, in much of Africa pregnant women, even during their last few months of pregnancy, remain active (see Fig. 8). The basal metabolic

37

rate (BMR) usually increases during pregnancy, which again raises energy requirements. Thus, most women in Africa need more energy when they are pregnant.

There is little doubt that abortions, miscarriages and stillbirths are commoner in women who are poorly nourished than in those who are adequately nourished. Dietary deficiencies probably also increase the risk of producing a malformed foetus. Severe malnutrition reduces fertility and therefore the likelihood of conception. A severely malnourished woman ceases to menstruate. This is clearly a natural device to stop the loss of nutrients in the menstrual flow, and to protect the woman from the rigours of pregnancy and childbirth. Nevertheless, there is little evidence of lack of fertility among the less severely malnourished, who form the majority in Asia and parts of Africa.

The weight of the infant at birth is influenced by maternal nutrition. Low birth weights can be expected in malnourished mothers. A modest increase in energy intake during pregnancy tends to increase the birth weight of the infant. Infants with a low birth weight have a much greater risk of dying. In Africa many girls have their first child while they are very young and immature. This is an added strain since they then need extra nutrients for the growth both of their own body and that of the foetus.

Anaemia is widespread in Africa, especially among pregnant women. This is largely because of the low absorption of iron from vegetables and cereals, and is aggravated when parasitic disease is present.

All pregnant women should attend a clinic at regular intervals for antenatal examination. Their haemoglobin level should be checked. Practical advice should be given regarding diet, taking into account what foods are locally available and what the mother can afford. It is useless to tell her to eat 200 grams of meat per day to ensure an adequate protein intake if she has no money to buy it, or if a beast is slaughtered only once a month in the village. A person running an antenatal clinic should be familiar with what local foods are available and are regularly eaten, and their nutritive value. Foods rich in protein, iron, calcium, and vitamin A are especially important during pregnancy.

In areas where anaemia is prevalent, pregnant women should be advised to take iron medicinally. This can be in the form of a ferrous sulphate tablet (200 mg) given three times a day. It is particularly important that this be taken during the last half of pregnancy. Vitamin supplements should be provided only if there is a special reason for doing so.

In areas where it is known that vitamin A deficiency is prevalent, cod-liver oil or multivitamin tablets can be prescribed. Sometimes medicinal folate (a B vitamin) is needed in addition to iron.

38

7. NUTRITION AND BREAST-FEEDING

Nutrition during lactation

During the delivery of an infant under hospital conditions, a woman may lose up to 1 litre of blood. The majority of women in Africa have their babies at home, and the persons assisting with the delivery may not know how to minimize blood loss. During the weeks after delivery the mother must replace the blood lost. The protein, iron, and other nutrients contained in the blood must be supplied in her diet.

At the same time, she begins to lactate. First colostrum, and, within a few days, milk are secreted by the breasts. Breast-feeding in Africa commonly continues for over a year, and not infrequently for 2 years. At about 8 months of age, the infant may often be receiving almost 1 litre of milk from its mother's breast.

One litre of milk provides 750 calories and contains the following:

Carbohydrate	70	g
Fat	46	g
Protein	13	g
Calcium	300	mg
Iron	2	mg
Vitamin A	480	µg
Thiamine	0.2	mg
Riboflavin	0.4	mg
Niacin	2	mg
Vitamin C	40	mg

As will be explained later, humans do not absorb all the nutrients they eat. Similarly, the conversion of nutrients in food to nutrients in breast milk is not entire. A lactating woman, therefore, in addition to the normal requirements, needs extra food to replace both the blood lost at delivery and the above nutrients she is providing as milk for her infant.

There is a widely held belief that the composition of breast milk varies enormously. This is not so. Human breast milk has a fairly constant composition, and is little affected by the diet of the mother. The carbohydrate, protein, fat, calcium and iron contents do not change much even if the mother is short of these in her diet. But a mother whose diet is deficient in thiamine, vitamin A and vitamin C produces less of

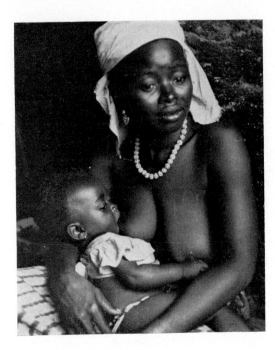

FIGURE 9. African women are usually good breast-feeders.

these in her milk, and, with thiamine at least, this can lead to a deficiency disease in her infant (infantile beriberi, see page 96).

Again contrary to some beliefs, the milk in both breasts has the same composition. Frequently mothers, or more often grandmothers, think that the milk from one breast is not good, and, much to the disadvantage of both mother and infant, only one breast is ever used. In general the effect of very poor nutrition on a lactating woman is to reduce the quantity rather than the quality of breast milk.

Lactating mothers should be encouraged to attend a clinic with their babies during the months after delivery. At the clinic both mother and baby should be examined. The mother should have her haemoglobin level checked and also her weight. Medicinal iron in the same quantities as recommended during pregnancy should be given. The mother should be given advice on feeding a mixed diet.

The baby should be examined at each visit. A satisfactory gain in weight is the best way of judging the adequacy of the diet of the infant. The mother should be given every encouragement to continue breast-feeding for as long as possible. On the whole, mothers in Africa are excellent breast-feeders, and failure of lactation is uncommon (see Figs. 9,

40

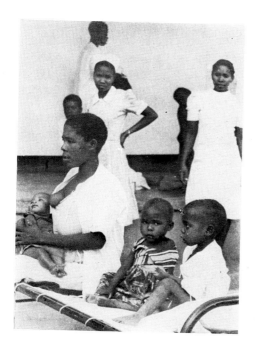

FIGURE 10. The African child shows good growth and satisfactory weight gain while he gets adequate breast milk. The three children shown here are siblings. The baby on the left is 9 months old, breast-fed and of good size for his age. The other two children, aged 3 and 5 years, are small and not well-grown.

10). Mothers should be advised not to give the infant any supplementary foods until he is 4 months of age, provided that he is gaining weight normally and appears healthy. After this, supplementary foods should be introduced by the sixth month at latest, but breast-feeding should still continue. Supplements should include foods rich in iron (without which the infant may become anaemic), foods containing vitamin C, and foods that provide good quantities of calories for growth and for the extra energy that the infant now expends. As soon as the supply of breast milk is reduced, it is vitally important to include other protein-rich foods in the infant's diet.

At clinics, time is often wasted in teaching mothers how to breast-feed a baby properly. These lessons are frequently given by women who have not themselves had children, and who try to pass on western textbook ideas about breast-feeding. Insistence on burping, on timing of feeds, on breast support, on positioning the baby for the feed are out of place in Africa. Breast-feeding is not a complicated, difficult procedure. The low rate of successful breast-feeders in North America and Western Europe is an indication of how poor western-style teaching has been. Not that there is any great harm in burping, or frequently cleansing the nipples, or feeding every 4 hours for 15 minutes, but all these strictures have had the effect of giving breast-feeding a magical, mythical aura, and this has had grave psychological effects which have often resulted in failure of lactation.

Failure of lactation in a person of the lower socioeconomic group in Africa is a tragedy of considerable importance. Usually fresh cow's milk is unavailable. The price of full-cream powdered milk is so high as to make it impossible for most persons to use it in the correct quantities. The cost of feeding a 4-month-old baby solely on one of the standard whole milk products sold for infant feeding was KSh 130 (approximately US$18) per month at Nairobi prices in 1978. This is far too much for unskilled workers who may earn only KSh 300 (US$40) per month and for farming families whose cash income is often less than KSh 100 (US$14) per month. Even if the parents could afford to buy whole-cream powdered milk and a bottle with a teat, the chances of the baby surviving would be small.

Bottle-feeding

Bottle-feeding can be quite successful in a well-equipped house with an electric or gas stove, a refrigerator, and running water. However, these are not available in 95 percent of African households. It is almost impossible for a busy woman in a hut where cooking is done over an open fire and water is drawn several miles away to properly clean, sterilize, and prepare bottle-feeds for a baby. In these circumstances the chances of the bottle-fed infant dying of gastrointestinal infection or marasmus are very high.

For this reason it is deplorable to see the cult of bottle-feeding taking a grip on Africa. The immigrant community is largely to blame. What it does has often been regarded as sophisticated if not superior. Commercial companies have not been slow to exploit a potential market. Many vernacular newspapers and other media carry advertisements for one or more proprietary milk preparations for infant feeding. The advertisements imply that bottle-feeding is superior to breast-feeding, and they often include a picture of a well-dressed, contented mother bottle-feeding a fat, happy baby. The background may be a solid modern home, implying that it is sophisticated and less troublesome and in some way superior to bottle-feed a baby. The advertisement may stress the nutrients added to the milk powder without mentioning that no nutrients need to be added to breast milk for the first few months of lactation. This type of advertising has now spread to the cinema where short items show "how easy and how good" it is to bottle-feed with such-and-such a product. For the majority of Africans, however, bottle-feeding is a difficult, unnecessary and thoroughly bad practice.

Breast-feeding versus bottle-feeding

The famous paediatrician Paul György said "Cow's milk is best for baby cows and human breast milk is best for human babies". No one can deny the truth of that statement. However, science and industry have combined to produce milk products which mimic breast milk and contain nutrients in quantities fairly similar to those in breast milk. There is no adequate proof that breast-feeding is nutritionally vastly superior to bottle-feeding with these products for those who can afford them and who live in modern conditions. Nevertheless, no one would argue that these milk products or that the milk of other mammals are superior to human breast milk for infants. It is therefore strongly recommended that women breast-feed rather than bottle-feed unless there is some good reason for not doing so.

The advantages of breast-feeding over bottle-feeding include: the ready availability and convenience of breast-feeding; the adequacy of nutrients in breast milk; the lower chance of it leading to infant obesity; the economic benefits for the family and the nation (breast milk is the only low-cost, high-protein food of animal origin readily available); the good mother-child relationship fostered by breast-feeding; the immunity conferred by the globulins and other constituents in breast milk; the reduced likelihood of developing diarrhoea; and the contraceptive effect of breast-feeding.

Until fairly recently it was considered an old wives' tale that breast-feeding helped prevent pregnancy. There is now good evidence to show that, although it is not a reliable contraceptive method in itself, breast-feeding prolongs average birth intervals by 5 to 8 months. This is due to a hormonal effect that delays the return of ovulation. Also, in some societies, women who are breast-feeding do not have sexual intercourse, or have it less frequently than non-lactating women. In many countries, the wider spacing of children resulting from breast-feeding is perhaps having a greater influence on the rate of population increase than the pill or IUD.

Breast-feeding has advantages everywhere, and it is now recognized that for about two thirds of the world's population bottle-feeding of infants is highly undesirable. In many instances placing an infant on a bottle may be tantamount to signing its death certificate. Bottle-feeding is responsible for a vast amount of childhood illness and deaths. In many developing countries bottle-feeding is the cause of more deaths than is cancer — yet vast sums are spent on cancer research, journals and text-books are devoted to tumours, while research on breast-feeding is limited and the literature on the subject rather scanty.

Why is it that bottle-feeding is such a serious public-health problem for infants in developing countries and for the infants of the poor every-where? There are two main reasons:

Overdilution leads to marasmus. Bottle-feeding frequently leads to undernourishment, then nutritional marasmus and often death in infants in poor communities. The commercial products available for bottle-feeding are relatively expensive in terms of prevailing incomes in devel-oping countries. As a result the family often purchases too little of the milk, or formula, and overdilutes the mixture in the bottle. The infant may be given the correct number of feedings and the recommended volume of liquid, but each feeding is too low in its content of calories and other nutrients. The result is a slow but inevitable development of nutritional marasmus. In Tanzania in 1963, the cost of adequately feeding a 6-month-old infant was equivalent to half the minimum wage in that country. No family can afford to spend over half of its income on food for the youngest member. It was also estimated that in continental Tan-zania with about 10 million persons the production of human milk was approximately 40 million gallons per year. Its value, if substituted with powdered cow's milk or milk formula, would have been US$22 million per year. This sum considerably exceeded the total budget of the Ministry of Health in 1963. The relative cost has not altered much since then.

Contamination leads to diarrhoea. Poor hygiene with bottle-feeding is a major cause of gastroenteritis and diarrhoea in infants, since milk is a good vehicle and culture medium for pathogenic organisms. Breast-fed children in developing countries have a much lower incidence of di-arrhoea. Mortality statistics from most poor communities show that gastrointestinal infections are the single largest cause of infant deaths. The paediatric wards of tropical hospitals are full of babies dying of this disease. It is extremely difficult to provide uncontaminated bottle-feeding: when the family water supply is a ditch or a well, contaminated with human excrement (and few households in developing countries have their own safe supply of running water); when household hygiene is poor and the home environment is contaminated by flies and faeces; when there is no refrigerator or other safe storage place for a previously pre-pared formula; when there is no turn-on stove, and when each time the bottle needs to be sterilized or water needs to be boiled, someone has to gather fuel and light a fire; when there is no suitable equipment for cleaning the bottle between feeds or when the bottle used is a cracked and almost

44

uncleanable soft-drinks bottle; and lastly when the mother has little knowledge of hygiene and does not even understand the fundamental germ concept of disease.

Why is there a trend to bottle-feeding and why is it spreading so rapidly in developing countries, especially in the urban areas? In some instances this is due to the break-up of the extended family, the emancipation of women and the need of women to take their place in the work force, although in some countries it is accepted practice to encourage working women to nurse their babies at their place of employment, and provide facilities for it.

Among the factors influencing the decline in breast-feeding in developing countries are western influence, medical advice and advertising.

Western influence. North American and European mothers, whose behaviour and dress are a potent influence in many poor societis, seldom breast-feed. Western society has developed a sort of breast culture in which the female breast has become a dominant sex symbol — it is accentuated in books, by the media and in women's clothes. At the same time it has become an object of prudery. Yet in many African countries women expose their breasts for feeding in public quite naturally. It is accepted that infants be breast-fed in public places, as was once also the case in the United States and Europe. Nevertheless a belief has developed that it is superior, chic and sophisticated to bottle-feed. As a result of such beliefs breast-feeding tends to be regarded as a "primitive" practice and the bottle becomes a status symbol.

Medical advice. In some countries the medical profession must take a large share of the blame for the decline in breast-feeding. In many hospitals infants are placed on the bottle while their mothers are still in the obstetric wards, and few obstetricians or paediatricians take positive steps to encourage breast-feeding. In some instances the manufacturing companies have employed African women, dressed them in white uniforms like nurses, and sent these "milk nurses" into hospitals and clinics to promote their milk product. Often free tins of milk powder are given to mothers after delivery. The mother may use this for a few weeks and only then realize its high cost, but because she has not been breast-feeding her milk may have dried up. She has no alternative but to carry on the expensive and dangerous practice of bottle-feeding. In many hospitals advertisements for breast-milk substitutes are found on the walls of out-patient departments, wards and doctors' offices.

Advertising and marketing of products for bottle-feeding. This is possibly the single most important reason for the rapid decline in breast-feeding in developing countries in recent years. The advertising onslaught is terrific, the message powerful, the profit to be made high, as is the resultant human suffering. The manufacturers also use aggressive marketing techniques and often try to influence members of the medical and health profession to advise their childbearing patients to bottle-feed.

African governments should give serious thought to passing legislation to ban this type of advertising, and to control the merchandising of these products. In Guinea-Bissau infant formulas are now not available for purchase by the general public except with a medical prescription.

Lactation failure

There are a few instances, however, where a mother genuinely has difficulty in breast-feeding. She should, if possible, be admitted to hospital and placed in a ward where other women are successfully breast-feeding. She should be examined for any physical reason for not being able to breast-feed. She should be given plenty of fluids, including milk. All these are mainly psychological inducements aimed at encouraging the resumption of lactation.

If breast-feeding remains unsuccessful, then she should be taught to feed milk to the baby either with a cup and spoon, or with a feeding bowl. Some means should be found to provide her with adequate fresh milk or full-cream milk powder if she cannot afford to buy it, which will usually be the case. A cup and spoon are easier to keep clean than are a bottle and teat. The infant should attend the clinic regularly. This method of feeding also applies to the infant of a mother who dies in childbirth. It is then desirable to admit to hospital with the child whichever female relative is to be responsible for feeding him. An alternative is to find a lactating relative or friend to breast-feed the infant and to act as a wet nurse.

Failure of lactation or death of the mother after the infant is 4 months of age calls for a different regime. The child can be fed a thin gruel (or *uji*) of whatever is the local staple food. To this should be added adequate quantities of full cream or, failing that, dired skim milk powder. If the latter is being used, it would be advantageous to provide some extra fat in the infant's diet. A relatively small quantity of groundnut, sesame (simsim), cottonseed, red palm, or other edible oil will markedly increase the energy intake without adding too much to the bulk. If milk or milk powder is not available then any of the highly protein-rich foods, such as legumes, eggs, ground meat, fish or poultry, may be used.

46

8. NUTRITION OF THE CHILD

First 6 months of life

Provided that the mother has adequate breast milk, breast-feeding alone with no added food or medicinal supplementation is all that is needed for the normal infant during the first 4 or 5 months of life.

The child should be examined regularly at the clinic. If the child was premature or one of twins, then his iron reserves may be small, and either an iron mixture or iron-rich food should be introduced before he reaches 6 months of age. Under certain conditions, and especially with diarrhoea, it will be necessary to give the child regular sips of water. Since contaminated water or utensils can easily transmit disease, both should always be boiled shortly before use.

On the whole, African children show good growth during their first 6 months of life, equal to or better than that of children in highly developed countries. Up to this age breast-fed children have considerable natural immunity to many infectious diseases.

Weaning period

During the weaning period semi-solid and then solid foods are introduced, while breast-feeding continues. From 6 months to 12 months, it is highly desirable that breast-feeding should continue and that the child should get as much milk as possible from his mother. At about 4 or 5 months of age, other foods should be introduced to the diet of the infant if his growth and health are to be normal.

It has been mentioned that breast milk is relatively deficient in iron and that the infant's store of iron is sufficient only until about 6 months of age. From 6 months to 12 months, the normal infant may be expected to gain between 2 and 3 kg in weight. Unless he drinks very large quantities of breast milk, he will need food to provide extra energy, protein, iron and vitamin C for his growth.

The energy can usually be obtained from a gruel or *uji* of whatever is the local staple food, but the quantity and bulk of the *uji* can profitably be reduced if some edible oil or fat-containing food is also eaten. If the staple is a cereal such as maize, millet, or rice, it will also provide a useful quantity of protein, but if it is banana, or a root such as cassava or yam, it will supply very little protein. In either case, but especially in the latter, it is vitally important to provide extra protein-rich foods. If these are not available, then dried skim milk, which may be obtainable free of cost at a clinic, should be added. Milk or milk powder can usefully be added to a number of foods eaten by the child. A fresh egg beaten into the gruel while it is simmering in the pan is another simple way of providing excellent protein for the toddler. Meat or fish if cut up finely after cooking will also provide protein of good quality.

Animal-protein products may not be available, or may be too expensive for a family budget. Legumes such as beans, peas, lentils, cowpeas and groundnuts are good sources of protein and should be added to the diet of the child. These can be ground or crushed before or after cooking. A thick soup made of crushed groundnuts is an excellent and highly nutritious food for the toddler. Although large quantities of beans cause flatulence and sometimes abdominal pains in adults, there is no reason why they should cause any great trouble in young children, given in moderate quantities, and provided the bean skin is removed.

The above foods, as well as providing energy and protein, will also provide some iron. Additional iron and the required vitamin C can best be obtained from edible green leaves, which also contain carotene. A small portion of whatever green vegetable (amaranth, cassava leaves, uncultivated leaves) is being cooked for the family should be removed from the pot before the rest of the family eat. It should be chopped up and added to the gruel of the infant or toddler, or fed to him separately. This will provide good quantities of iron, carotene (vitamin A) and vitamin C.

Carotene and vitamin C can also be obtained from fruit. Ripe papayas and mangoes are excellent and usually most acceptable to young children. Vitamin C can alternatively be provided in citrus fruits (e.g., oranges), or in other fruits (e.g., guavas). A 6-month-old child need not have a whole orange at one sitting. Instead, when the mother or father eat one, they can squeeze out a tablespoonful or two of juice and feed it to the infant.

Gradually, as the child gets more teeth, he can be put onto a more solid diet. By the age of 2 years, breast-feeding will usually have ceased and the child be completely weaned.

The period from 6 months to 2 years is of paramount importance nutritionally. The mother should take the child regularly to a clinic if one is available. The happiness, the general appearance and the weight of the child are the best general indication of adequate nutrition. The use of a weight chart to help the mother follow the growth of the child is described in Chapter 19. Many children of this age in Africa do not grow at the rate they should, and some develop protein-energy malnutrition. Those who fail to grow may be heading toward this disease, which may strike them during the next year or two. It may be precipitated by an attack of a complaint such as measles, whooping cough or diarrhoea, or by events of psychological importance, such as the sudden removal of the child from the mother (see p. 113).

During this period the child becomes more active. He begins to crawl and later walk, he picks objects up and puts them in his mouth, he burrows his hands in the moist earth, he even paddles with his brother in the local streams. These activities may expose him to some of the common ailments of Africa — hookworm, schistosomiasis, malaria, ascariasis, dysentery, etc.

He may also develop one of the infectious diseases of childhood. All the diseases from which he was partially protected during his early life may strike him now, and affect his nutritional status.

The mother responsible for feeding a toddler who is no longer breast-feeding must keep in mind that the child:

— Needs a variety of foods, as great or greater than that given to any other member of the family;
— Is growing rapidly and needs extra protein-rich foods;
— Has few teeth, and requires soft food;
— Has a relatively small appetite and intake capacity and needs more frequent meals than older persons;
— Requires clean food and clean utensils to avoid infection;
— Must as far as possible be protected from communicable diseases;
— Should have the love, affection, and personal attention of his mother both for his mental and, indirectly, his physical well-being. Attention from the father and other members of the family will also contribute to his development and well-being.

The proper feeding of a toddler requires time and patience. Special utensils or equipment are not necessary, but a sieve or strainer is useful. Adult foods can be chopped up and forced through a strainer into a cup or onto a plateful of gruel for the child. A strainer can readily be made if not available. Otherwise, various foods can be crushed before cooking using a pestle and mortar, which are found in most households. Some foods are better crushed with a wooden spoon or with a fork. Some examples of suitable foods for young children are given in Chapter 36.

Preschool child aged 2 to 5 years

During the early part of this period, the problems faced by the child are similar to those mentioned for the weaning period. The child remains in danger of developing protein-energy malnutrition, nutritional anaemia or xerophthalmia. He is still not able to cope fully with an adult diet. The problems must be faced in the way mentioned above.

In the latter half of this period, the child can eat a diet similar to the rest of the family. He may not, however, like peppery, hot, or spicy foods. Often the protein-rich portion of the family meal is a stew or sauce to which chilies, onions and curry powder have been added. Consequently, the child may eat just the carbohydrate portion of the diet because it is the only bland part of the meal; this may be a cause of malnutrition.

Another problem with children in this age group is that they often have the lowest priority at the table. The men may eat first and take most of the beans, meat and other nutritious portions of the family meal. The small child, less forceful than his older brothers and sisters, may thus get practically none of these portions.

A child between 2 and 5 years of age is growing rapidly and may need to be fed more frequently than the older members of the family to obtain the recommended allowances shown in Table 1 of Appendix 1. Parents should understand the needs of the child and see that the right foods are available, prepared in ways palatable to him, and that he gets his fair share. They will thus require nutrition education. A number of recipes of dishes suitable for young children are given in Chapter 36.

School-age child

The vast majority of children at school in Africa are attending primary schools. Most are at day schools, few of which provide a midday meal. In rural areas, the school is often some kilometres from the parents' home. The child frequently has to leave home early and walk a considerable distance to school. Often there is no breakfast for him at home before he leaves, he gets no meal at school, and returns for his first and sometimes his only meal of the day late in the afternoon.

The nutritional needs of a schoolchild are high (see Table 1 in Appendix 1). The adolescent child has proportionately higher requirements of most nutrients than does the average adult. It is practically impossible for him to obtain adequate quantities of the right foods from one, or even two, meals a day. It is highly desirable that he eat some food before going to school, and some food at school.

Food before going to school. Many mothers are not prepared to rise before dawn to spend the considerable length of time necessary to light a fire and prepare a hot meal for the child before he sets off for school. Therefore, if no hot breakfast is available, some fruit, cold cooked po-

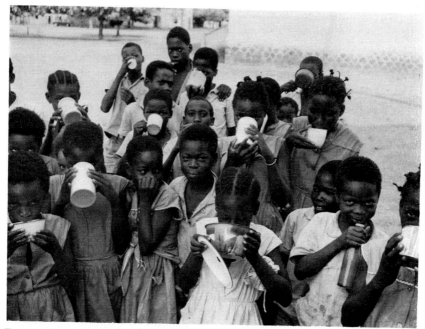

FIGURE 11. A midday meal (or snack) at day schools is very important. Following the introduction of a protein-rich snack at this school in the Ivory Coast, the children grew more, their haemoglobin improved, and absenteeism was reduced.

tatoes or cassava, or even cold porridge or *ugali* should be left over from the previous day for the schoolchild to eat before he leaves home in the morning.

Food eaten at school. This may consist of a midday school meal or a snack taken to school.

MIDDAY SCHOOL MEAL. A midday school meal is the ideal, and should provide reasonable amounts of the nutrients most likely to be missing or short in the home diet. In Africa it might therefore often include some protein-rich food, some food containing vitamins A and C, and some calcium-containing foods. A whole-grain cereal as the basis, with added milk powder and a side dish of legumes with green leaves, is excellent. There are very many possibilities, depending on what foods are locally available. A number of suitable school diets are given in Chapter 37.

School meals are beneficial because they often supply much-needed nutrients: they can form the basis for nutrition education; they are a good way of introducing new foods; and they prevent hunger and malnutrition (see Fig. 11).

Further nutrition education can be carried out as an extracurricular project. A school vegetable garden or orchard can provide valuable extra nutrients for the midday meal. Poultry keeping, small animal production (rabbits, guinea pigs, pigeons, etc.), and the building of a fish pond are all projects suitable in certain areas. They are educative and can provide food for a school meal (see Fig. 12).

A midday school meal might be provided by the government or local authority as part of the educational system, and could be paid for from the normal school fees. Alternatively, a midday meal system might be started and paid for from special fees collected from the pupils daily, weekly, or per term. Local organizations might provide certain food items free or at low prices for school feeding, thus reducing the overall cost.

The cost of school feeding can be reduced by local self-help efforts performed by villagers, parents' committees and pupils. This may fit in well with the "Harambee" (independence) spirit in Kenya or be a part of services provided by an *ujamaa* village in Tanzania. For example, a small kitchen shelter can be built on a self-help basis. Instead of hiring a paid cook, a rota of mothers can take turns doing the cooking. Pupils can collect firewood at week-ends. School lunches need not be hot, since cold meals are just as nutritious. However, it should be stressed that the provision of a midday school meal must not detract from the parents' responsibilities to provide a good diet for schoolchildren at home.

SNACK TAKEN TO SCHOOL. In the absence of a school lunch, parents should send their children to school with some food to be eaten at midday. There is a real difficulty in finding suitable foods, however. The problem is similar to that of providing a cold breakfast, so the various foods suggested for this can equally be used for a midday snack. The sort of food taken will vary according to what is available locally. Possibilities include a few bananas, cooked whole cassava, sweet or ordinary potatoes roasted in their skins, fruit, tomatoes, roasted maize on the cob, roasted ground-nuts, coconuts, cold grilled fish, smoked cooked meat, hard-boiled eggs, a calabash of sour milk, or some bread.

Many schools above primary level are boarding schools. These usually provide three meals a day, and the menu should be based on recommendations made to the school by someone with dietetics training. Suitable school diets are mentioned in Chapter 37. Occasionally schools plead lack of money as an excuse for an inadequate diet. School meals need not be luxurious, but should be balanced and provide all the nutrients necessary for growth and health. The child on an inadequate diet will not only fail to grow properly, but may also develop anaemia and other signs of malnutrition, and will not be able to concentrate on or benefit fully from the education being provided for him.

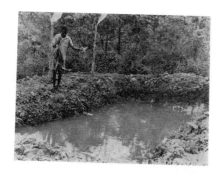

FIGURE 12. Examples of school food-production projects.

Fishpond

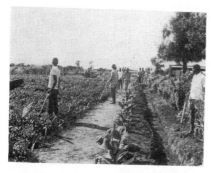

School garden

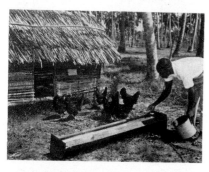

Poultry keeping

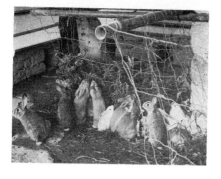

Rabbit keeping

II. BASIC NUTRITION

9. THE FUNCTIONS OF FOOD

"We are what we eat" is a statement frequently used to illustrate that the composition of our bodies is dependent in large measure on what we have consumed.

Before considering the different foods necessary to nurture that very complicated mechanism, the human body, it is desirable first to learn something of the chemical composition of the body. The body of an adult has the following approximate chemical composition:

Element	Percentage of body weight
Oxygen	65
Carbon	18
Hydrogen	10
Nitrogen	3.0
Calcium	1.5
Phosphorus	1.0
Potassium	0.55
Sulphur	0.25
Sodium	0.15
Chlorine	0.15
Others (including magnesium, iron, manganese, copper, iodine)	0.55

These substances occur mainly in the form of water, protein, fats, mineral salts and carbohydrates, in the following percentages:

Item	Percentage of body weight
Water	63
Protein	17
Fats	12
Minerals	7
Carbohydrates	1

The body is built up from these five constituents and vitamins in food. Food seves mainly for growth, energy, and body repair and maintenance. Food also provides enjoyment and stimulation since eating and drinking are among the pleasures of life. Truly food nourishes both the body and soul. Even if technology could produce a perfect diet in terms of content, it would probably lack, for example, the aroma and flavour of a curry, or the stimulating taste of hot coffee.

A convenient, though incomplete, classification of dietary constituents is given below.

Item	Use
Carbohydrates	Fuel energy for body heat and work
Fats	Fuel energy and essential fatty acids
Proteins	For growth and repair
Minerals	For developing body tissues and for metabolic processes
Vitamins	For metabolic processes
Water	To provide body fluid and to help regulate body temperature
Spices and flavourings	To add enjoyment to eating
Indigestible and unabsorbable particles	To form a vehicle for other nutrients, add bulk to the diet, provide a habitat for bacterial flora, and assist proper elimination.

The general term for all the chemical processes carried out by the cells of the body is "metabolism". Chief among these processes is the oxidation (combustion, or burning) of the food with the production of energy (like a motor-car engine burning petrol to produce energy for it to move). In most forms of combustion, be it in the motor car or in the human, heat is produced as well as energy.

Traditional physics has taught that energy can neither be created nor destroyed, a law of nature that, though not completely correct (as the conversion of matter to energy in a nuclear reactor shows), is still true in most instances. Energy for the body comes from food, and, in the absence of food, can be produced only by the breakdown of body tissues. All forms of energy can be converted to heat energy. Thus, for example, it is possible to measure the heat produced by burning a litre of petrol. Food energy can also be and is expressed as heat energy. The unit of measurement used has been the (large) Calorie or kilocalorie (this is one thousand times the small calorie used in physics). The Calorie is defined as the heat necessary to raise the temperature of 1 litre of water from 14.5 to 15.5°C. It is a unit of measurement in the same way that litres and pints are measures of quantity, and metres and feet are measures of length. Nowadays the joule is being introduced in place of the Calorie (see conversion tables, Appendix 4), but there are still discussions going on as to which is the most useful unit to express food energy.

The human body requires energy for all bodily functions, including the maintenance of body temperature and the continuous action of the heart and lungs. Energy is also needed for breakdown, repair, and the building of tissues. These are metabolic processes. The rate at which these functions are carried out while the body is at rest is the basal metabolic rate (BMR). This varies with sex, age, body size, diseases, such as goitre, and many other factors.

The average human burns energy at his BMR only when at complete rest. All ordinary movements require additional energy, and physical work, of course, more still.

An average day may involve the following energy expenditure:

	Activity	Calories
Sleep:	8 hours of rest in bed, at a BMR of 1 Calorie per minute i.e., $8 \times 60 \times 1$	480
Light work:	8 hours of, say, herding cattle, at 2.5 Calories per minute, i.e., $8 \times 60 \times 2.5$	1 200
Other:	8 hours of sitting and minor activities, at 2 Calories per minute, i.e., $8 \times 60 \times 2$	960
	Total	2 640

If, instead of 8 hours of light work, the person in this example did 5 hours of herding and 3 hours of heavy work hoeing hard ground at 4 Calories per minute, then his output of energy would be:

	Activity	Calories
Sleep:	8 hours of rest in bed, at a BMR of 1 Calorie per minute	480
Light work:	5 hours of, say, herding, at 2.5 Calories per minute	750

Hard work: 3 hours of, say, hoeing, at 4 Calories per minute   720

Other: 8 hours of sitting and minor activities, at 2 Calories per minute   960

                                                    Total   2 910

Now consider what happens to the individual undertaking the activities mentioned in the first example if he gets exactly 2 640 Calories in his food: his weight will be steady, and he will be functioning normally. However, if he then undertakes the activities in the second example, and eats no extra food, his weight will gradually drop, because he will have to burn up his fuel reserve — which forms part of his own body. He would fairly soon, however, begin to limit his activities in order to stop this process. He would therefore probably work less hard at hoeing, so that instead of burning 4 Calories per minute, he might use only, say, 3.2 Calories; he would also tend to be tired at the end of the day, and might well increase his period of complete rest (at 1 Calorie per minute) by reducing the period of minor activities. He would therefore have reduced his calorie requirements to 2 646 as follows:

Activity		**Calories**
Sleep:	10 hours of rest in bed, at a BMR of 1 Calorie per minute	600
Light work:	5 hours, at 2.5 Calories per minute	750
Hard work:	3 hours of less hard work, at 3.2 Calories per minute	576
Other:	6 hours of sitting and minor activities, at 2 Calories per minute	720
	Total	2 646

This is just an example. In most instances when people increase their output of energy, including work, they feel more hungry, and they increase their consumption of their staple food, be it rice, millet, maize, or anything else.

The energy requirements of a human being are affected by:

Body size. A small person needs less energy than a large person.

Basal metabolic rate. It has already been mentioned that the BMR varies and that it can be affected by factors including disease of the thyroid gland.

Activity. The more physical work or play performed, the more energy is required.

Pregnancy. A woman requires extra energy to develop, and to carry the additional weight of, the foetus.

Lactation. The lactating mother needs additional energy to produce energy-containing milk for the suckling baby. The relatively long duration of breast-feeding among most Africans results in a large proportion of women requiring extra energy.

Age. Infants and children need more energy for growth and activity than older persons, in whom the need for energy is reduced because there is a decline in activity and because the BMR is usually lower.

Climate. In a warm climate, such as that in most of tropical Africa, less energy is necessary to keep the body at its normal temperature than in cold climates.

10. CARBOHYDRATES, FATS AND PROTEINS

Carbohydrates

The main source of energy for most Africans is derived from carbohydrate in the food they eat. Carbohydrates constitute by far the greatest portion of the African diet, as much as 80 percent in some cases. This is nearly twice the 45 to 50 percent of carbohydrates in the diets of many people in industrialized countries. Carbohydrates are compounds containing carbon, hydrogen and oxygen in the proportions 6:12:6. They are burned during metabolism to produce energy, liberating carbon dioxide (CO_2) and water (H_2O). In the human diet carbohydrates are provided mainly in the form of starches and the various sugars.

58

CARBOHYDRATES

Monosaccharides	Disaccharides	Polysaccharides
e.g., Glucose	e.g., Sucrose (table sugar)	e.g., Starch
Fructose	Lactose	Glycogen (animal starch)
Galactose	Maltose	Cellulose

The simplest carbohydrates are the monosaccharides, or simple sugars. These simple sugars can pass through the wall of the alimentary tract without being changed by the digestive enzymes. The three commonest are glucose, fructose, and galactose. Glucose, sometimes also called dextrose, is present in fruit, sweet potatoes, onions and other plant substances. It is the substance into which many other carbohydrates such as the disaccharides and starches are converted by the digestive enzymes. Glucose is oxidized in the production of energy and heat with the liberation of carbon dioxide, which is exhaled in breathing. Because glucose is the sugar in blood, it is the obvious choice for an energy-producing substance for persons being fed intravenously. Glucose dissolved in sterile water is frequently used for this purpose, usually in concentrations of 5 or 10 percent.

Fructose is present in honey and some fruit juices. Galactose is the monosaccharide that is formed, together with glucose, when digestive enzymes act on lactose, the sugar in milk.

The disaccharides, though fairly simple sugars, need to be converted by the body into monosaccharides before they can be absorbed from the alimentary tract. Examples of disaccharides are sucrose, lactose and maltose. Sucrose is the scientific name for table sugar (i.e., the kind that is used, for example, to sweeten tea). In Africa it is most commonly produced from sugar cane. It is also present in beets, carrots and pineapple. The disaccharide present in human and animal milk is lactose. It is much less sweet than sucrose. Maltose is found in germinating seeds.

The polysaccharides are chemically the most complicated carbohydrates. They tend to be insoluble in water, and only some can be used by human beings to produce energy. Examples of polysaccharides are starch, glycogen and cellulose. Starch, the polysaccharide found in cereal grains and also in root foods such as potatoes and cassava, is an important source of energy for man. Starch is carried in these foods as granules which, when heated, rupture and liberate the starch. This occurs during cooking. Glycogen is the polysaccharide made in the human body, and is sometimes known as animal starch. The process of glycogen formation is the reverse of the digestive action on some other polysaccharides. Thus starch from cassava is broken down in the intestines to form monosaccharide molecules. This monosaccharide passes to the bloodstream; surplus monosaccharide molecules are fused together in numbers to form a new polysaccharide, glycogen, as follows:

Starch $\longrightarrow$ monosaccharide $\longrightarrow$ energy $+ CO_2 + H_2O$

Surplus starch $\longrightarrow$ monosaccharide $\longrightarrow$ glycogen.

Glycogen is usually present in the muscle and liver, but not in large amounts. Any of the digestible carbohydrates when consumed in excess of body needs are converted by the body into fat and laid down as adipose (or fat) tissue.

Cellulose is a third polysaccharide; it is the fibre of green plants, and is also present in wood. The human alimentary tract cannot break down cellulose and utilize it to produce energy. Some animals such as cattle have micro-organisms in their intestines which break down the cellulose and make it available as an energy-producing food. Cellulose forms much of the bulk and roughage evacuated in human faeces.

It is now recognized that the high fibre content of most traditional African diets may be an important factor in the prevention of certain diseases that appear to be much more prevalent in people consuming the low-fibre diets common in developed countries. Fibre, by inducing the rapid passage of materials through the intestine, may be a factor in the control of diverticulitis, appendicitis, haemorrhoids and also possibly coronary heart disease.

Fats

In African diets, fats usually provide fewer calories than carbohydrates do, perhaps only 8 or 10 percent of the total calories. In most industrialized countries, the proportional intake of fat is much higher; in the United States, for example, an average of 40 to 45 percent of the energy derives from fat.

Fats, like carbohydrates, contain carbon, hydrogen and oxygen. They are insoluble in water, but soluble in such chemical solvents as ether, chloroform and benzene. The term "fat" is used here to include all fats and oils that are edible and occur in human diets. These range from

60

fats such as butter, which at cool room-temperatures are solid, to ground-nut or cottonseed oils which at similar temperatures are liquid. In some terminology the word "oil" is used for those materials that are liquid at (European) room temperature and fat for those that are solid.

Fats consist mainly of triglycerides, which can be split to form glycerol and fatty acids. This action is achieved in the human intestine by enzymes known as lipases. These are present primarily in the pancreatic and intestinal secretions. Bile salts from the liver emulsify the fatty acids making these more soluble in water.

The fatty acids are divided into two main groups: the saturated and the unsaturated (including both polyunsaturated and mono-unsaturated). Saturated fatty acids have the maximum number of hydrogen atoms that their chemical structure will permit. All fats and oils eaten by man are mixtures of saturated and unsaturated fatty acids. Broadly speaking, fats from land animals (i.e., meat fat, and butter) contain more saturated fatty acids than do those of vegetable origin. Fats from plant products and to some extent from fish have more unsaturated fatty acids, particularly those called polyunsaturated. But there are exceptions: for example, coconut oil has a large amount of saturated fatty acid.

These groupings of the fats have caught public attention, especially since excess intake of saturated fats appears to be one of the causative factors in arteriosclerosis and coronary heart disease. This finding is of minor importance in Africa, where most people consume relatively little fat, and of this the bulk contains mainly unsaturated fatty acids. In the minority who do have a high fat intake, such as the Samburu of Kenya and the Masai of Tanzania, diseases attributed to an increased intake of these fats are rare. Degenerative diseases, possibly due to a high fat intake, are said to occur in Senegal and possibly some other African countries. The precise role of fat in the causation of these diseases has yet to be fully elucidated. It seems likely that the amount of exercise taken and the consequent lack of adipose tissue found in Africans on a high-fat diet, compared with the sedentary existence and the obesity of their counterparts in developed countries, may be significant factors. Coronary heart disease is becoming more common among affluent Africans who are consuming westernized diets, are more likely to be obese, and who may also smoke cigarettes. Western diets tend to be high in cholesterol, which, together with saturated fats, may raise serum cholesterol levels.

Fat is desirable in a diet to make it more palatable. It also yields about 9 Calories per gram, more than twice as much energy as carbohydrates and proteins do (about 4 Calories/gram), and can therefore reduce the bulk of the diet. A person doing very heavy work, especially in a cold climate, may require as many as 4 000 Calories a day. It is then highly desirable that a good proportion of this energy should come from fat; otherwise the diet would be very bulky. Fats form a vehicle for the fat-soluble vitamins, which will be discussed later. Three of the unsaturated fatty acids have been termed "essential fatty acids". These are the polyethenoid acids, which are important in the synthesis of the important human hormones, the prostaglandins. Experiments with animals and studies in man have shown definite skin and growth changes in the absence of these fatty acids and there is no doubt that they are essential for the nutrition of individual cells and tissues of the body. Thus fats, and even specific types of fat, are essential to health. However, practically all diets provide the small amount required.

Fat deposited in the human body serves as a reserve fuel. It is an economic way of storing energy, because, as mentioned earlier, fat yields about twice as much energy, weight for weight, as does carbohydrate or protein. Fat is present beneath the skin as an insulation against cold, and it forms a supporting tissue for many organs such as the heart and intestines. It must be remembered that the fat in the body is not necessarily derived from fat that has been eaten. A cow or pig gains fat on a mainly carbohydrate diet. Similarly, excess calories from a carbohydrate source such as maize, cassava or banana can be converted into fat in the human body.

Proteins

Proteins, like carbohydrates and fats, contain carbon, hydrogen and oxygen, but they also contain nitrogen and often sulphur. They are particularly important as nitrogenous substances, and are necessary for the growth and repair of the body. The main structural constituents of the cells and tissues of the body are proteins. The greater portion of the substance of the muscles and organs (other than water) is protein. Although proteins can yield energy, their main importance is rather as an essential constituent of all cells. It should be remembered that all cells, from time to time, may need replacement.

Just as complicated carbohydrates such as starches break down into simple monosaccharides like glucose, and fats break down into fatty acids, so proteins break down during digestion to form amino acids. These are organic compounds containing the amino group NH_2.

Plants are able to synthesize amino acids from simple inorganic chemical substances. Animals do not have this ability: all the amino acids necessary for building their protein come from consumption of plants or animals. As the animals we eat originally derived their protein from plants, all amino acids in human diets have come ultimately from this source. Animals have differing abilities to convert one amino acid into another; in the human this ability is very limited. Conversion occurs mainly in the liver. If this ability to convert one amino acid into another were unlimited, then the question of protein deficiency and of the protein content of diets would become simple and straightforward. It would merely be a matter of supplying enough protein irrespective of the quality or amino-acid content of that protein.

There are a large number of amino acids, about 20 of which are common in plants and animals. Of these, eight have been found to be essential for the adult human, and have thus been termed "essential amino acids". They are: phenylalanine, tryptophan, methionine, lysine, leucine, isoleucine, valine and threonine. A ninth amino acid, histidine, is required for growth and is essential for infants and children; it may also be necessary for tissue repair.[1] Each protein in a particular food is a mixture of amino acids, and can contain up to all eight of the essential ones.

Proteins consumed in the diet undergo a series of chemical changes in the gastrointestinal tract. The physiology of this is complicated: pepsin and rennin from the stomach, trypsin from the pancreas, and erepsin from the intestines hydrolyse proteins into their component amino acids. The amino acids are absorbed into the bloodstream from the small intestine, travel to the liver, and from there all over the body. How each cell in the body, with its need for certain amino acids, competes for its requirements, especially when there is a deficiency, is unknown. Any surplus amino acids are stripped of the amino (NH_2) group, which goes to form urea in the urine, leaving the rest of the molecule to be transformed into either fat or the polysaccharide, glycogen.

There is no true storage of protein in the body, as there is with fat and, to a small extent, glycogen. However, there is now little doubt that a well-nourished individual has sufficient protein accumulated to be able to last several days without replenishment and still remain in good health. Similarly, it has been shown in Africa that malnourished subjects can accumulate protein without any gain in body weight.

It is important to know the quantities of total protein a food contains, the individual amino acids present in the protein and the quantities and proportion of essential amino acids included.

Much is now known about the individual proteins present in various foods and about their amino acid content. A number of different methods have been devised to give these proteins a chemical "score" with which

---

[1] The other known amino acids are: glycine, alanine, serine, cystine, tyrosine, aspartic acid, glutamic acid, proline, hydroxyproline, citrulline and arginine.

to define their value. However, a chemical scoring system tends to give values that may appear exact, but are not, because some proteins, especially those of vegetable origin, are not utilized completely. For this reason, the chemical scores of various proteins are not given here.

Nevertheless, the value of any given protein does depend on its constituent amino acids. Some are better than others, and these are said to have a higher biological value. Proteins such as albumin in egg and casein in milk contain all the essential amino acids in good proportions, and are superior to such proteins as zein in maize, which contains little tryptophan or lysine, and the protein in wheat, which contains only small quantities of lysine. While the protein in milk or egg is nutritionally better than that in maize or wheat, it is not true to say that the last two are worthless. Although deficient in certain amino acids, they do contain many other important amino acids. With maize and wheat the deficiency can be overcome by providing other foodstuffs containing the missing amino acids. It is therefore possible for two foods, each with poor protein, together to form a good protein mixture.

As an example, if the letters A, B, C, D, E, F, G, H represent the eight essential amino acids, a given food might contain amino acids A, B, C, D, E in good amounts, but if eaten as the only source of protein would provide an unsatisfactory diet, since it lacks amino acids F, G and H. This could be put right either by eating some very good protein (such as that of milk or eggs) that contains all eight essential amino acids, or by eating a less good protein that contains, for example, amino acids F, G and H.

This illustrates that people, especially those on a diet deficient in animal protein, require a *variety* of foods of vegetable origin, not just one staple food. In many African diets, pulses or legumes such as groundnuts, beans and cowpeas, though themselves short of sulphur-containing amino acids, supplement the cereal proteins, which are often short of lysine. A mixture of foods of vegetable origin especially if *taken at the same meal* can serve as a substitute for animal protein.

FAO has produced tables showing the contents of essential amino acids in different foodstuffs (FAO, 1970); from tables such as these it can be seen which foods best supplement each other. It is also necessary, of course, to ascertain the total quantity of protein and amino acids in any food.

This raises the difficult question as to what is the desirable or the necessary protein intake for a human being. Proteins are necessary:

— For growth and development of the body;
— For body maintenance, and the repair and replacement of worn out or damaged tissues;

64

— To produce metabolic and digestive enzymes;

— As an essential constituent of certain hormones, such as thyroxine and insulin.

The minimum quantity of nitrogen excreted by an average adult is approximately 3 g/day, representing about 19 g of protein. However, for various reasons, rather more protein than this is required in the daily diet. A Joint FAO/WHO Expert Committee (FAO, 1973) recommended a daily requirement of 0.55 g of milk or egg protein per kilogram of body weight for an adult male. Since people eat mixed diets and do not get all their protein from milk or eggs, an adjustment must be made for protein quality. For example, if the proteins in the diet have a value of say 70 percent of egg or milk protein, the daily requirement will be

$$0.55 \times \frac{100}{70}, \text{ or } 0.8 \text{ g/kg body weight.}$$

Children's needs for protein are higher than adults' because they are growing; infants may need 2 g of milk protein per kilogram body weight per day, and rather less — 1.2 g — in early childhood. If the protein in a mixed diet is only 70 percent of the quality of milk protein a 7-kg infant may require 21 g and a 25-kg child 50 g of protein per day.

A pregnant woman needs an additional supply of protein to build up the foetus inside her. Similarly, a lactating woman needs extra protein, because the milk she is secreting contains protein. Thus, a woman secreting, for example, 0.8 litre of milk will be providing 13 g of protein for her infant, and she herself will require this extra amount in her diet. As her protein conversion is never 100 percent, it is inevitable that a considerable amount of extra protein is required per day. In Africa it is common for women to breast-feed their babies for as long as 2 years. Thus some African women need extra protein for 2 years and 9 months for every infant.

Although in most of Africa the intake of protein is low, there are some peoples who have an exceptionally high protein intake. The Masai, living on a diet consisting mainly of milk and meat and occasionally fresh animal blood, may consume 200 g or more of protein daily. This high-protein diet seems to be well tolerated, and in fact the physique of the Masai is generally superior to that of their neighbours. This may be due to genetic and ethnological reasons, as well as the nutritional ones.

Low-protein diets are nearly all of predominantly vegetable origin, and are not usually consumed as a matter of choice. Most Africans like animal products, but these are less freely available, more difficult to produce and store, and more expensive than most vegetable products. A diet low in meat, fish, or dairy products tends to be unattractive, but in countries where most people are poor such diets are the rule.

As is pointed out elsewhere, infections lead to an increased loss of nitrogen from the body. This has to be replaced by proteins in the diet. Therefore children and others who have frequent infections will have protein needs above those of healthy persons. This fact must constantly be borne in mind, for in Africa many children suffer an almost continual series of infectious diseases; they may frequently get diarrhoea, and they may harbour intestinal parasites.

11. MINERALS

Minerals have a number of functions in the body. They are present as salts in body fluids, where sodium, potassium and chlorine play a physiological role in maintaining osmotic pressure; they form part of the constitution of many tissues (e.g., in bones, calcium and phosphorus combine to give rigidity to the whole body); they are present in body acids and alkalis (e.g., chlorine of hydrochloric acid in the stomach); and they are an essential constituent of certain hormones (e.g., iodine in the thyroxine produced by the thyroid gland).

The principal minerals present in the human body are calcium, phosphorus, potassium, sodium, chlorine, sulphur, copper, magnesium, manganese, iron, iodine and fluorine.

Phosphorus is so widely available in plants that a shortage of this element does not present a nutritional problem. Potassium, sodium and chlorine are easily absorbed, and are more important than phosphorus from a physiological point of view. Sulphur is consumed by humans mainly in the form of sulphur-containing amino acids, and so sulphur deficiency, if it occurred, would be linked with protein deficiency. Copper and magnesium have not been widely reported in Africa. There is no definite evidence concerning the function of manganese in human metabolism. Zinc deficiency may contribute to a rare form of dwarfing found in the Near East. The minerals that are of most importance in human nutrition are thus calcium, iron, iodine and fluorine, and only these will be discussed here.

Calcium

The body of an average-sized adult contains about 1 250 g of calcium. Most of this is present in the bones and teeth, where it is combined with phosphorus as calcium phosphate, forming a hard substance that gives the body rigidity. However, although hard and rigid, the skeleton of the body is not the unchanging structure it appears to be. In fact, the bones are a cellular matrix, and the calcium is taken up by the bones and given back to the body continuously. The bones therefore serve as a reserve supply of this mineral.

Calcium is present in the serum of the blood in small but important quantities, usually about 10 mg per 100 ml of serum. A reduction in this amount causes the condition of tetany (not to be confused with the disease tetanus, an infection with the tetanus bacillus), described on page 107.

There are also about 10 g of calcium in the extracellular fluids and soft tissues of an adult body.

All the calcium in the body, except that inherited from the individual's mother, normally comes from food consumed. It is especially necessary to have adequate quantities of calcium during growth, for it is at this stage that the bones are being developed.

FIGURE 13. Distribution of milk. Here milk is being sold by cattle owners for distribution to areas short of milk.

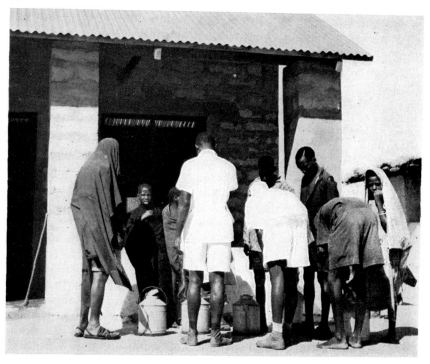

The foetus in the uterus of its mother has its nutritional requirements completely satisfied, for, nutritionally, the unborn child is truly parasitic. The mother, if her diet is poor in calcium, draws extra supplies of this mineral from her bones. Similarly an entirely breast-fed infant, provided that the volume of milk is sufficient, will get adequate calcium, since, contrary to popular belief, the composition of human milk is very constant, especially with regard to calcium. Breast milk, even of an undernourished mother on a diet very low in calcium, provides approximately 30 mg calcium per 100 ml. A lactating mother secreting 1 litre will thus be losing 300 mg of calcium per day.

As soon as the child stops receiving adequate quantities of breast milk, it faces for the first time the possibility of a shortage of calcium, and in many African diets this possibility becomes a reality. Cow's milk is a very rich source of calcium, richer than human milk. However, all too often cow's milk is unavailable to African children (see Fig. 13). A litre of human milk contains 300 mg of calcium, while a litre of cow's milk contains 1 200 mg. This difference arises because a cow has to provide for its calf, which grows much more quickly than a human infant, and needs extra calcium for the hardening of its fast-growing skeleton. Similarly the milk of other domestic animals has a higher calcium content than human milk.

A child (or even a baby) drinking large quantities of cow's milk excretes any excess calcium; the extra does no harm, but does not increase the growth rate beyond the optimal.

Calcium content of various milks utilized in Africa

Source	Content (mg/100 ml)
Human	30
Cow	120
Camel	120
Goat	130
Sheep	200

Milk products such as cheese are also rich sources of calcium, but cheese is not yet important in African diets, even in areas of high milk production. Small saltwater and freshwater fish such as sardines and sprats supply good quantities of calcium since they are usually eaten whole, bones and all. Small dried fish known as *dagaa* in Tanzania and *kapenta* in Zambia may commonly be eaten and add useful calcium to the diet.

Vegetables and pulses provide some calcium. Although cereals and roots are relatively poor sources of calcium, they often supply the major portion in tropical diets by virtue of the quantities consumed. The calcium content of drinking water varies from place to place.

The absorption of calcium is variable and generally rather low. It is related to the absorption of phosphorus and other main mineral constitutents of the bones. Vitamin D is essential for the proper absorption of calcium, and protein also is believed to assist. The reverse is true of phytic acid in certain cereals and oxalic acid in fruits and vegetables such as spinach and rhubarb which can inhibit calcium absorption. It is thus difficult to state categorically the human requirements of calcium.

The following are recommended levels of calcium intake, based on suggestions by WHO and FAO:

Category	Daily intake (mg)
Adults	400 - 500
Children	400 - 700
Pregnant and lactating women	1 000 - 1 200

Disease or malformation due primarily to a dietary deficiency of calcium is rare. Rickets in children and osteomalacia in adults are both usually due to a deficiency of vitamin D, which in turn causes a calcium deficiency. A low calcium intake does not appear related to dental caries.

It is possible that the small stature of some peoples in Africa and elsewhere may be due in part at least to generations of a low intake of calcium. However, those peoples are also often deficient in protein and other nutrients and are afflicted with many diseases that inhibit proper development.

Iron

The average iron content in a healthy adult is only about 3 g, yet this relatively small quantity is vitally important. Iron deficiency is a leading cause of ill health in many parts of the world, including much of Africa.

The major portion of this iron is present in the red blood cells linked to a protein in the form of a pigment called haemoglobin. Haemoglobin serves to carry oxygen from the lungs to the cells of the body and return carbon dioxide to the lungs. If the body, for some reason, has insufficient iron, then the amount of haemoglobin will be reduced and anaemia will follow.

A small quantity of iron is present in the chromatin and other molecules in the cells, and in a compound present in muscle called myoglobin. This iron is not released, even in an anaemic patient.

However, the healthy body does have a small store of iron, perhaps 0.5 g in all, present as the compound ferritin in the liver, spleen and bone marrow. This can be utilized in a subject who becomes deficient in iron.

It is important to remember that iron is not an element that is used up or destroyed in the body. The body is very economical and conservative in the use of iron. That which is released when the red blood cells are old and broken down is taken up again and used for the synthesis of new red cells. Similarly, red blood cells destroyed by malaria parasites shed their iron, but this too is utilized again. In normal conditions, less than 1 mg of iron is lost to the body each day.

It follows that a healthy man's nutritional needs for iron are very small unless there has been a loss of blood, while women must make good the blood lost at menstruation and during childbirth, and they must meet the additional requirements of pregnancy and lactation. However, in considering man's dietary needs for iron, it must be kept in mind that only about 10 percent of the iron present in cereals, vegetables and pulses, excluding soybeans, is absorbed. Absorption from other foods is somewhat higher: 30 percent from meat, 20 percent from soybeans. Absorption increases when there is increased formation of haemoglobin to replace losses through haemorrhage, etc., and during growth and pregnancy. Phytic acid and an excess of iron salts may hinder iron absorption because insoluble iron salts are formed.

Human milk contains only about 2 mg of iron per litre, and cow's milk half this amount. The foetus, however, is supplied with a store of iron by the pregnant mother. This store, together with the small quantity of iron contained in breast milk, should be sufficient to last until the infant is 6 months of age. In much of Africa, babies are breast-fed for well over a year, and unless iron-containing foods are introduced at about the age of 6 months to supplement this milk diet, iron deficiency anaemia is likely to develop (see p. 144). Similarly, with premature infants and multiple births, the infant's iron store is reduced and iron deficiency anaemia is much more likely to occur.

It can be seen that women have increased needs for iron at various stages of their lives. Women need more during pregnancy, both to provide the iron for the blood and tissues of the foetus and a store of iron for the infant. A woman loses perhaps 750 ml of blood containing iron during childbirth, and this needs replacing. As mentioned above, the lactating woman secretes 2 mg of iron per litre of milk, and a menstruating woman loses some iron-containing blood each month.

70

Growing children increase not only their body size, but also their blood volume. Therefore, they too have relatively large iron requirements.

It is suggested that a daily allowance of 5-9 mg/day is appropriate for adult men and post-menopausal women. Women should receive 14-28 mg/day during reproductive life (see Table 1 in Appendix 1).

Iron is present in most foodstuffs, but its content in plants tends to vary according to the soil. The richest plant sources are green leaves, followed by vegetables and fruits. Man's main supply usually comes from his staple food, be it cereals, starchy roots or animal products. Cereals contain almost twice as much iron as starchy roots, while fish and meat contain good quantities, especially in the internal organs such as the liver, heart and kidneys.

Upon examination, very few diets appear to be grossly deficient in iron, even if they are poor in most other respects. However, it must be remembered that, as pointed out above, only a portion of the iron in the diet is absorbed. There are many factors that determine how much iron in a food can be utilized by the human body.

The foregoing should not lead to the belief that it is rare for people to become deficient in iron. In much of Africa it is commoner for people to harbour parasites than not to do so. Hookworm is present in 75 percent of the population of some areas; and schistosomiasis (bilharzia) is extremely common. Most of these parasites cause loss of blood. Another common source of loss among the poorer people is ulcers and accidental wounds. Whenever blood is lost, iron is also lost, and if it is not replaced, iron-deficiency anaemia will result.

Iodine

The body of an average adult contains about 20-50 mg of iodine, of which about 8 mg are present in the thyroid gland. Iodine is essential for the formation of thyroxine, the hormone secreted by this gland.

A lack of iodine in the diet causes an enlargement of the thyroid gland, a condition known as goitre (see Fig. 14). The thyroid gland is situated in the lower front part of the neck. There are other causes of goitre though undoubtedly iodine deficiency is by far the commonest cause of endemic goitre (see also page 139).

In certain areas where goitre was common, the authorities added iodine to the salt, which gradually freed these areas from the complaint. The substance usually added to salt has in the past been potassium *iodide*, but another form, potassium *iodate*, is more stable and better in hot, humid climates.

As elsewhere in the world, goitre is common in Africa in certain plateau areas far from the sea. For example, an investigation carried out by the author in the Njombe area of Tanzania revealed that 75 percent of the population had some enlargement of the thyroid.

Iodine is widely present in rocks and soils, but the quantity in different plants varies according to the soil in which they are grown. Iodine tends to get washed out of the soil, and throughout the ages a considerable quantity has flowed into the sea.

Sea fish, and most vegetables grown near the sea are useful sources of iodine. However, it is not meaningful to list the iodine content of foodstuffs because of the large variations in this content.

Fluorine

Fluorine is found mainly in the teeth and skeleton. Traces of fluorine in the teeth help to protect them against decay. Some fluorine consumed during childhood becomes a part of the dental enamel and thereby makes the enamel more resistant to the weak organic acids formed from foods that adhere to or get stuck in between the teeth. This greatly reduces the chances of decay or caries developing in these teeth. Recent studies suggest that fluorine may also help strengthen bone, particularly later in life, and thus inhibit the development of osteoporosis.

The main source of fluorine for most human beings is the water they

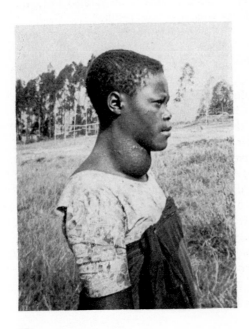

FIGURE 14. Goitre in an adolescent girl. There are patterned marks over the swelling where cuts have been made and traditional medicine applied.

72

drink. If this contains about 1 part of fluorine per million, then it will supply adequate fluorine for the teeth. There are many waters, however, that contain much less than this. Fluorine is present in bone, and consequently small fish that are consumed whole are a good source. Tea has a high content of fluorine, but it does not appear to be utilized by humans. No other foods contain much fluorine. If the fluorine content of drinking water in any locality is below 0.5 part per million, dental caries will probably be more prevalent than if the concentration were higher.

In some countries where the content of fluorine in the water is less than one part per million, it has now become the practice to add fluorine to the water supply. This is strongly to be recommended, but is only practicable for large piped-water supplies. In Africa, where most people do not get their water in this manner, it is not a feasible proposition. The addition of fluorine to salt is being investigated as a means of supplying this mineral nutrient to people who do not have access to a fluorinated water supply. Fluorine does not prevent dental caries, but can reduce the incidence by 60 to 70 percent.

It is possible to have too much fluorine, however. An excessively high intake of fluorine during childhood causes a condition known as dental fluorosis, in which the teeth become mottled as a result of too

FIGURE 15. Fluorotic teeth.

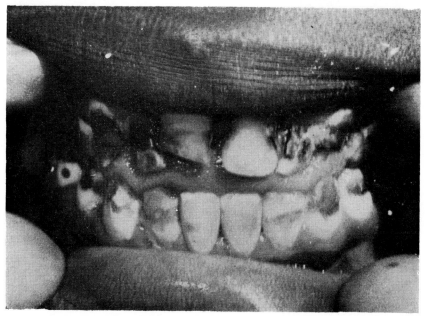

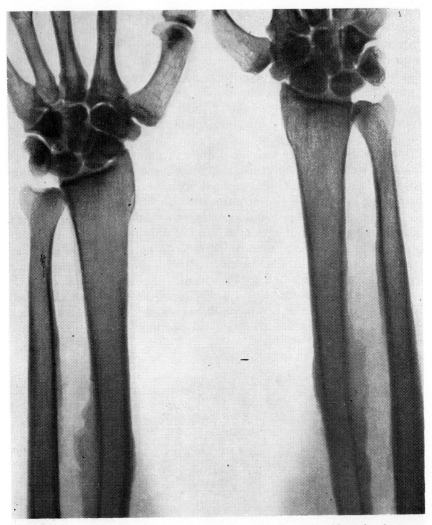

FIGURE 16. X-ray of the forearms of a person with fluorosis. Note the denseness of the bones and the calcification between them.

much fluorine in the water supplies (see Fig. 15). In some parts of Africa natural waters contain over four parts per million of fluorine. Very large intakes of fluorine cause bone changes with sclerosis, calcification of muscle insertions, and exostoses. A survey carried out by the author in Tanzania revealed a high incidence of fluorotic bone changes (as shown by X-ray) in older subjects (see Fig. 16) who normally drank water containing over 6 parts per million of fluorine.

74

12. VITAMINS

Vitamins are organic substances present in minute amounts in foodstuffs and necessary for metabolism. They are grouped together not because they are chemically related or have similar physiological functions, but because, as their name implies, they are vital factors in the diet. Moreover, they do not fit into the other categories — carbohydrates, fats and proteins — of nutrients.

When vitamins were first being classified, each was named after a letter of the alphabet. Subsequently, there has been a tendency to drop the letters in favour of chemical names. This is justified when the vitamin has a known chemical formula, as with the main vitamins of the B group. Nevertheless, it is advantageous to include them under one heading since, though not chemically related, they do tend to occur in the same foodstuffs. In this book only vitamin A, five of the B group of vitamins (thiamine, riboflavin, niacin, vitamin B_{12} and folic acid), vitamin C and vitamin D will be described. Other vitamins known to be vital to health include pantothenic acid (a deficiency of this may cause the "burning feet" syndrome mentioned on p. 148), biotin (vitamin H), para-amino-benzoic acid, choline, vitamin E and vitamin K (antihaemorrhagic vitamin). These vitamins are not described here for one or more of the following four reasons: deficiency is not known to occur under natural conditions in man; a deficiency is extremely rare in even grossly abnormal diets in Africa; disease due to a lack of them occurs only following some other disease process that is adequately described in textbooks of general medicine; the role of the vitamin in human nutrition has not yet been elucidated.

In any event none of these vitamins are important from the point of view of workers studying nutrition as a community-health problem in Africa. Those wishing to learn more about them are referred to texbooks of general medicine or more detailed texbooks of nutrition. A summary of the conditions associated with vitamin deficiencies is given in the table.

VITAMIN A (RETINOL)

History. Vitamin A was discovered in 1913 when research workers found that if the only form of fat present in the diet of certain laboratory animals was lard (made from pork fat), then the animals stopped growing, whereas if the diet remained exactly the same, except that butter was supplied instead of lard, the animals grew and thrived. It was clear that there was some substance in the butter that was not present in the lard.

The chief vitamins — a summary

Vitamin	Chemical name	Associated conditions	Units
A	Retinol	Night blindness, xerophthalmia, follicular keratosis, keratomalacia	µg (formerly IU)
B₁	Thiamine (aneurin)	Beriberi	mg
B₂	Riboflavin	Cheilosis, angular stomatitis, and other lesions of tongue and skin	mg
PP	Niacin (nicotinamide, nicotinic acid)	Pellagra	mg
B₆	Pyridoxal, pyridoxamine, pyridoxine	Convulsions	mg
B₁₂	Cyanocobalamin	Pernicious anaemia	µg
—	Folacin (folic acid, pteroglutamic acid)	Macrocytic anaemia, sprue	mg
C	Ascorbic acid	Scurvy	mg
D	Calciferol	Rickets, osteomalacia	IU
—	Pantothenic acid	"Burning feet" syndrome	mg
K		Haemorrhagic disease	mg

This substance seemed to be necessary for the health of the animals, even though both diets contained adequate quantities of carbohydrates, fats, proteins and minerals. Further animal experiments showed that egg yolk and cod-liver oil contained the same vital food factor, which was named vitamin A.

It was later established that many vegetable products had the same nutritional properties as the vitamin A present in butter. The reason was that they contained a yellow pigment called carotene, which can be converted to vitamin A in the human body.

Properties. In its pure crystalline form, Vitamin A or retinol[1] is a very pale yellow-green substance. It is soluble in fat but insoluble in water, and is found only in animal products.

Carotenes, which, as mentioned above, act as provitamins or precursors of vitamin A, are yellow substances that occur widely in plant

---

[1] Retinol is the chemical name of the alcohol derivative and is used as the reference standard.

76

substances. The yellow colour of the carotene may in some foodstuffs be masked by the green plant pigment, chlorophyll, which often occurs in close association with it. There are several different carotenes; one of these, beta carotene, is the most important source of vitamin A in African diets. The conversion of these substances into vitamin A takes place in the walls of the intestines. Because losses occur in the conversion it is accepted that 1 μg of absorbed beta carotene has the biological activity of 0.5 μg of retinol. Only about one third of the beta carotene in food is absorbed and available. Therefore 1 μg of beta carotene in food is equivalent to about 1/6 μg of retinol. Intestinal diseases such as dysentery, and infections with common intestinal parasites such as roundworm, which are common in the tropics, tend to reduce the ability of the body to convert carotene into vitamin A (see below).

The liver acts as the main store of vitamin A in the human and most other vertebrates, which is why there is a high content of this vitamin in fish-liver oils.

Vitamin A is an important component of the visual purple of the retina of the eye, and if vitamin A is deficient, the ability of the eye to see in dim light is reduced. This is called "night blindness".

The biochemical basis for the other lesions of vitamin A deficiency has not been fully explained. The main change in pathological terms is a keratinizing metaplasia which is seen on various epithelial surfaces. Vitamin A appears to be necessary for the protection of surface tissue. Deficiency results in various conditions including follicular keratosis in the skin and pathological drying of the eye leading to xerophthalmia and sometimes keratomalacia. These conditions are described later (see p. 103).

Units. Vitamin A used to be measured in international units (IU), but amounts are now usually stated in micrograms (μg) of retinol or retinol-equivalent. One international unit of vitamin A is equivalent to 0.3 μg retinol, or 0.55 μg retinyl palmitate.

Dietary sources. Vitamin A itself is found only in animal products; the main sources are butter, eggs, milk, liver and some fish. However, most Africans rely mainly on carotene for their supply of vitamin A. Many plant foods contain carotene; dark green leaves such as those of the amaranth (*mchicha*), sweet potato and cassava are much richer sources than the paler leaves of, for example, cabbage and lettuce. Various pigmented fruits and vegetables such as mangoes, papayas (see Fig. 17), tomatoes and carrots contain useful quantities. Yellow maize is the only cereal that contains carotene. Carotene is also present in small quantities in plantains and bananas as well as in yellow varieties of sweet

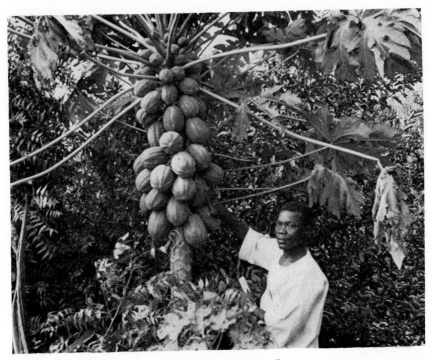

Figure 17. Papaya provides carotene and vitamin C.

potatoes. In West Africa much carotene is obtained from red palm oil, which is widely used in cooking. The cultivation of the very valuable oil palm is beginning to spread to other parts of the continent. Because of the high content of carotene, red palm oil is being used more and more as the cooking oil of choice in institutional diets.

Both carotene and vitamin A withstand ordinary cooking temperatures fairly well. However, a considerable loss of carotene takes place when green leaves and other foods are dried in the sun. This is often a traditional method of preserving wild leaves and vegetables in arid regions. Since serious disease due to vitamin A deficiency often occurs in these areas, it is important that better methods of preservation be established.

Factors influencing absorption and conversion. Even the most efficient intestine can only absorb and convert a portion of the carotene in the diet. If no animal products are consumed and the body relies entirely on carotene, allowances should be increased. Carotene is poorly utilized on a low fat diet, and diets deficient in vitamin A are very often deficient in fat. As mentioned above, intestinal diseases such as dysentery, coeliac

78

disease and sprue limit the absorption of vitamin A and the conversion of carotene. Furthermore, infants and young children do not convert carotene to vitamin A as readily as adults do.

Bile salts are essential for the absorption of vitamin A and carotene, and so persons with obstruction of the bile duct are likely to become deficient in vitamin A.

Hydrocarbon oils such as liquid paraffin markedly reduce carotene absorption. Liquid paraffin is widely regarded as a laxative that is simple and entirely safe. It is therefore frequently prescribed by medical personnel, or bought by the public in shops, to be taken daily for chronic constipation. If this is continued daily for many months it may lead to vitamin A deficiency.

Storage in the body. Vitamin A is stored mainly in the liver, and the amount present varies greatly. This store is important, for in many African diets foods containing vitamin A and carotene are available seasonally. If they are eaten in fairly large quantities during the wet season, for example, a store can be built up, which will help tide the person over at least a part of the dry season. The short mango season, for example, often replenishes the vitamin A stored in the liver of many African youngsters who spend their leisure hours foraging for this fruit.

Toxicity. Vitamin A, if taken in excess, causes undesirable toxic effects. Cases of this have occurred in West Africa due to a very high intake of red palm oil, and in some developed countries in children who have been given too much of a vitamin A preparation, such as halibut-liver oil. The most marked toxic effect is an irregular thickening of some long bones. This is usually accompanied by liver enlargement, skin changes and hair loss.

Human requirements. It is recommended that adults receive 750 μg of retinol per day; lactating mothers need 50 percent more, and children and infants less (see Table 1 in Appendix 1). It should be noted that these figures are based upon mixed diets containing both vitamin A and carotene. When the diet is entirely of vegetable origin larger amounts of carotene may be required because, as mentioned, the conversion from carotene to retinol is not very efficient.

THIAMINE (ANEURIN, VITAMIN B₁)

History. During the 1890s in Java (Indonesia), Dr Eijkman of the Netherlands noticed that when his chickens were fed on the same food as his beriberi patients, the chickens' legs became weak and they developed signs somewhat similar to those of beriberi. They also showed marked head retraction. The food of the beriberi patients was mainly highly polished rice. When he changed the diet of the chickens to whole-grain rice, they began to recover. He showed that there was a substance present in the outer layers and germ of the rice grain that protected the chickens from the disease.

Early in this century work done in a mental hospital in Malaysia showed that, under identical conditions, groups of persons fed polished rice developed beriberi, whereas those on unpolished rice did not. It was further demonstrated that the former group could be cured by putting them on a diet mainly of unpolished rice. Despite many attempts, it was only in 1926 that vitamin B₁, or thiamine, was finally isolated in crystalline form. It was synthesized 10 years later.

Properties. Thiamine is highly soluble in water. It resists temperatures of up to 100°C, but tends to be destroyed if heated above this (e.g., during frying in a hot pan or cooking under pressure). Thiamine has a rather loosely bound structure and is readily decomposed in an alkaline medium.

A large amount of research has been carried out on the physiological effects and biochemical properties of thiamine. This has shown that thiamine plays a very important role in carbohydrate metabolism in man. It is utilized in the complicated mechanism of the breakdown or oxidation of carbohydrate and the metabolism of pyruvic acid. The energy used by the nervous system is derived entirely from carbohydrate; a deficiency of thiamine leads to a shortage of energy, and lesions of the nervous tissues and the brain. It is because thiamine is concerned with carbohydrate metabolism that a person whose main supply of energy comes from carbohydrates is more likely to develop signs of thiamine deficiency. For this reason, thiamine requirements are sometimes expressed in relation to intake of carbohydrate.

Units. Thiamine has been synthesized in pure form and is now measured in milligrams.

Dietary sources. Thiamine is widely distributed in foods of both vegetable and animal origin. The richest sources are, however, cereal grains and pulses. Green vegetables, fish, meat, fruit and milk all contain useful quantities. With seeds such as cereals, the thiamine is present mainly in the germ and in the outer coats. Much is therefore liable to be lost during the milling of these products, as will be discussed later. Bran of rice, wheat or other cereals, and yeasts tend to be naturally rich in thiamine. Root crops, including cassava, are poor sources, the latter containing only about the same low quantity as polished rice. It is surprising that beriberi is not common among the many African peoples who live mainly on cassava.

Because it is very soluble in water, thiamine is liable to be lost from food that is washed too thoroughly or cooked in excess water, afterwards discarded. It is especially important that people on a rice diet use either just the amount of water that the rice will absorb in cooking, or use what is left over for making a soup or stew, for this water will contain thiamine and other nutrients.

Well-stored cereals and pulses maintain their thiamine for a year or more, but if attacked by bacteria, insects or moulds, the content of thiamine gradually diminishes.

Storage in the body. Thiamine is easily absorbed from the intestinal tract, but little is stored in the body. Experimental evidence indicates that man can store only enough for about 6 weeks. The liver, heart and brain have a higher concentration than the muscles and other organs.

A person on a high intake of thiamine soon begins to excrete increased quantities in the urine. The total amount present in the body is about 25 mg.

Human requirements. A daily intake of 1.0 mg of thiamine is sufficient for the moderately active man and one of 0.8 mg for a moderately active woman. Pregnant and lactating women may need more (see Table 1 in Appendix 1).

However, man's requirements of thiamine depend to a certain extent on his intake of carbohydrate. The figures in Table 1 of Appendix 1 are based on a recommended daily intake of 0.4 mg for every 1 000 calories. The disease beriberi, which is due mainly to a deficiency of thiamine, is discussed on p. 93.

RIBOFLAVIN (VITAMIN B₂)

History. Early work on the properties of vitamins in yeast and other foodstuffs showed that the antineuritic factors were destroyed by excessive heat, but that a growth-promoting factor was not destroyed in this way. This turned out to be riboflavin, which was later isolated from the heat-resistant portion. It was synthesized in 1935.

Properties. Riboflavin is a yellow crystalline substance. It is much less soluble in water than is thiamine, and is more heat resistant. It is destroyed more easily in acid than in alkaline solutions. The vitamin is sensitive to sunlight, and therefore foods such as milk may lose considerable quantities of riboflavin if left exposed. Riboflavin acts as a coenzyme concerned with tissue oxidation. In experimental animals, deficiency causes failure of growth, and also lesions, mainly of the skin and eyes. The possible role of riboflavin deficiency as a contributory factor in eye lesions including those of xerophthalmia has not been adequately investigated.

Units. Riboflavin is measured in milligrams.

Dietary sources. The richest sources are milk and its non-fat products, green vegetables, meat (especially liver), fish, and eggs. However, the main sources in African diets, which do not contain much of the above products, are usually cereal grains and pulses. Like thiamine, the quantity of riboflavin present is much reduced by milling and is lower in highly milled cereals than in lightly milled cereals. Similarly, starchy foods such as cassava, plantains, yams and sweet potatoes are poor sources.

Human requirements. Approximately 1.5 mg per day are ample for an average adult, but rather more may be desirable during pregnancy and lactation. Signs of riboflavin deficiency are frequently seen in many parts of Africa. The clinical signs are described on p. 152.

NIACIN (NICOTINIC ACID, NICOTINAMIDE, VITAMIN PP)

History. Just as the history of thiamine is linked with the disease beriberi, so the history of niacin is closely linked with the disease pellagra. Beriberi is associated with the Orient and a rice diet, pellagra with the Occident and a maize diet.

Pellagra was first attributed to a poor diet over 200 years ago by Casal. It was believed that pellagra might be due to a protein deficiency, because the disease could be cured by some diets rich in protein. Later it was shown that a liver extract almost devoid of protein could cure pellagra, and in 1926 Goldberger in the United States demonstrated that yeast extract contained a pellagra preventing (PP) non-protein substance. In 1937 niacinamide (nicotinic acid amide) was isolated, and this was found to cure "black tongue", a pellagra-like disease occurring in dogs.

Because pellagra was found mainly in those whose staple diet was maize, it was assumed that maize was particularly poor in niacin. It has since been shown that white bread contains much less niacin than maize. It is now known that the niacin in maize is not fully available because it is in a bound form.

82

The discovery that the amino acid tryptophan prevents pellagra in experimental animals just as niacin does complicated the picture until it was shown that tryptophan is converted to niacin in the human body. This work vindicated and explained the early theories that protein could prevent pellagra. It should be noted that zein, the main protein in maize, is very deficient in the amino acid tryptophan. This further explains the relationship between maize and pellagra. It has also been shown that a high intake of leucine, as occurs among sorghum-eaters, interferes with tryptophan and niacin metabolism and may cause pellagra.

Properties. Niacin is a derivative of pyridine. It is related to nicotine but, unlike the latter, it is non-toxic. Niacin is a white crystalline substance, soluble in water, and extremely stable. It has been synthesized. The main role of niacin in the body is in tissue oxidation.

Units. Niacin is measured in milligrams.

Dietary sources. Niacin is widely distributed in foods of both animal and vegetable origin. Particularly good sources are meat (especially liver), groundnuts, and cereal bran or germ. Like other B vitamins, the main source of supply in African diets tends to be the staple food. Wholegrain or lightly milled cereals contain much more than highly milled cereal grain. The starchy roots and plantains and milk are poor sources. Beans, peas, and other pulses contain amounts similar to most cereals. As stated earlier, the niacin present in maize does not seem to be fully utilizable.

Cooking, preservation, and storage of food cause little loss of niacin. However, like thiamine, niacin may be wasted in water discarded after cooking cereals, meat or any other niacin-containing food.

Human requirements. An adequate quantity for any person is provided by 20 mg per day. As indicated above, requirements are affected by the amount of tryptophan-containing protein consumed, and also by the staple diet (i.e., whether it is maize-containing or not).

Deficiency of the vitamin is prevalent in many parts of Africa; the disease associated with deficiency (pellagra) is discussed on p. 98.

VITAMIN B₁₂ (CYANOCOBALAMIN)

History. The disease pernicious anaemia, so named because it invariably used to be fatal, was known for many years before its cause was determined. In 1926 it was found that the patient improved if he ate raw liver. This led to the preparation of liver extracts which, when given by injection, controlled the disease.

In 1948 scientists isolated from liver a substance they called vitamin B_{12} which, when given in very small quantities by injection, was effective in the treatment of pernicious anaemia.

Properties. Vitamin B_{12} is a red crystalline substance containing the metal cobalt. It is necessary for the production of healthy red blood cells. A small addition of vitamin B_{12} or foods rich in it to the diet of experimental animals produces increased growth.

Units. Vitamin B_{12} is measured in micrograms (μg).

Dietary sources. Vitamin B_{12} is present only in foods of animal origin. It can also be synthesized by many bacteria. Herbivorous animals such as cattle get their vitamin B_{12} from the action of bacteria on vegetable matter in their rumen. Humans apparently do not obtain vitamin B_{12} by bacterial action in their digestive tracts.

Deficiency. Pernicious anaemia is not caused by a dietary deficiency of vitamin B_{12} but is due to the inability of the subject to utilize the vitamin B_{12} in his diet. In pernicious anaemia the red blood cells are larger than normal (macrocytic) and the bone marrow contains many abnormal cells called megaloblasts. This macrocytic or megaloblastic anaemia is accompanied by a lack of hydrochloric acid in the stomach (achlorhydria); later, serious changes in the nervous system take place. If left untreated, the patient dies.

Treatment consists of giving large doses of vitamin B_{12} by injection. When the blood characteristics have returned to normal the patient can usually be maintained in good health by receiving one injection of 250 μg of vitamin B_{12} every 2-4 weeks.

Vitamin B_{12} will also cure the anaemia accompanying the disease sprue. This is a tropical condition in which the absorption of vitamin B_{12}, folic acid and other nutrients is impaired.

The tapeworm, *Diphyllobothrium latum*, which man gets from eating raw or undercooked fish, lives in the intestines and has a propensity for removing vitamin B_{12} from the food of its host. This results in the development in man of a megaloblastic anaemia, which can be cured by injection of vitamin B_{12} and treatment to rid the patient of the tapeworm.

Other than in the above conditions deficiency of vitamin B_{12} is likely to occur only in those on a vegetarian diet. A deficiency causes anaemia and may produce neurological symptoms. The importance of vitamin B_{12} deficiency as a cause of megaloblastic anaemia in Africa is unknown, but is probably relatively small.

84

Human requirements. The human daily requirements of this vitamin are quite small, probably around 5 μg for adults usually, and 8 μg during pregnancy.

FOLIC ACID OR FOLATES (PTEROGLUTAMIC ACID)

History. In the 1930s Dr Lucy Wills discovered that the macrocytic anaemia commonly found among pregnant women in India responded to certain yeast preparations even though it did not respond to iron or any other known vitamin.

The substance present in the yeast extract that cured the macrocytic anaemia was at first called Wills' factor. Later (1946), a substance called folic acid, which had been isolated from spinach leaves, was found to have the same effect.

Properties. Folic acid is the group name given to a number of yellow crystalline compounds related to pteroglutamic acid. Diets deficient in folic acid cause chickens and monkeys to develop an anaemia in which the red blood cells are abnormally large (macrocytic). The folic acid present in foodstuffs is easily destroyed by cooking.

Units. Folic acid is measured in milligrams.

Dietary sources. The richest sources are dark green leaves, and liver and kidney.

Other vegetables and meats contain smaller amounts.

Deficiency. A deficiency leads to the development of macrocytic anaemia. Anaemia due to folate deficiency is the second most common type of nutritional anaemia after iron deficiency. The anaemia of sprue will respond to folic acid just as it will to vitamin B_{12}. However, although the blood picture will improve if folic acid is given to persons with pernicious anaemia, the nervous system symptoms will neither be prevented nor improved by it.

For this reason, folic acid should never be used in the treatment of pernicious anaemia except in conjunction with vitamin B_{12}.

The main therapeutic use of folic acid is in the treatment of nutritional macrocytic or megaloblastic anaemias of pregnancy and infancy, when a dose of 5 to 10 mg daily is recommended for an adult.

Human requirements. The recommended daily intake has been set at 200 μg for adults (FAO, 1974).

VITAMIN C (ASCORBIC ACID)

History. The history of vitamin C is associated with the disease scurvy in the same way that thiamine is linked with beriberi, and niacin with pellagra.

However, the history of scurvy goes back much further than either beriberi or pellagra. The disease was first recorded by seafarers making prolonged journeys. In 1497, Vasco da Gama, making his historical voyage from Europe around the southern tip of Africa to reach India, described scurvy among his crew.

It gradually became apparent that scurvy occurred only in persons who ate no fresh food. It was, however, not until 1747 that a Scotsman named Lind demonstrated that scurvy could be prevented or cured by the consumption of citrus fruit. This led to the introduction of fresh food, especially citrus products, as part of the ration of seafarers. Subsequently scurvy became much less common.

However, in the nineteenth century, scurvy began for the first time to occur among infants receiving a diet of the newly introduced preserved milk, instead of breast or fresh cow's milk. Although these preserved milks contained adequate carbohydrate, fat, protein and minerals, the infants still got scurvy because the milks were heated during processing, and the heat destroyed the vitamin C.

Properties. Ascorbic acid is a white crystalline substance that is highly soluble in water. It tends to be easily oxidized. It is not affected by light, but is destroyed by excessive heat, especially when in an alkaline solution.

Ascorbic acid is necessary for the proper formation and the maintenance of intercellular material. This is more easily understood if ascorbic acid is thought of as being an essential part of the substance that binds cells together, in the same way that cement binds bricks together. Thus, in a person suffering from ascorbic acid deficiency, the endothelial cells of the capillaries lack normal solidification. They are therefore fragile and haemorrhages take place. Similarly, the dentine of the teeth and the osteoid tissue of the bone are improperly formed. This cell-binding property also explains the poor scar formation and the slow healing of wounds manifest in persons deficient in ascorbic acid.

Ascorbic acid is believed to play some part in the formation of red blood cells. However, in experimentally induced vitamin C deficiency in man, anaemia has not been a feature, except following haemorrhages. Some scientists claim that very large doses of vitamin C both prevent and reduce symptoms of the common cold (coryza). This has not been verified, and it is not advisable to take very large doses of medicinal vitamin C for long periods of time.

86

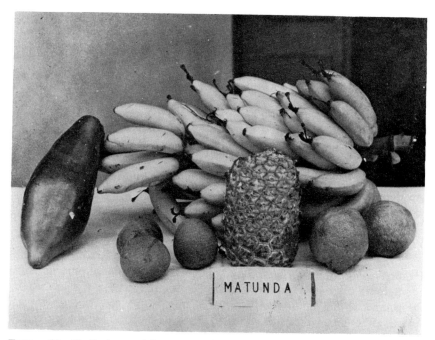

FIGURE 18. Fruits *(matunda)* are a good source of vitamin C, and many are also rich in carotene.

Units. Vitamin C is still sometimes referred to in terms of international units (IU). The original IU was defined as the amount of vitamin C present in 0.1 ml of lemon juice. As it has been isolated and synthesized, it is now preferable to measure it in terms of milligrams of the pure vitamin.

Dietary sources. The main sources of vitamin C in most African diets are fruits, vegetables and various leaves (see Fig. 18). In pastoral tribes milk is often the main source. Plantains or bananas are the one common staple food containing fair quantities of vitamin C (10 mg/100 g). Dark green leaves such as amaranth contain far more (100 mg/100 g) than the pale leaves of cabbage (41 mg/100 g), tomatoes (25 mg/100 g), or carrots (6 mg/100 g). The quantities found in tropical fruits such as papaya (50 mg/100 g) and mango (30 mg/100 g) are similar to those in most citrus fruits (40 mg/100 g). Guavas are extremely rich in vitamin C (200 mg/100 g). Wild fruit, including that of the baobab, and many non-cultivated leaves are often good sources, though many of these still need to be analysed to determine their exact ascorbic acid content. Root vegetables and potatoes contain small but useful quantities. Maize when eaten young provides some ascorbic acid, as do sprouted cereals and pulses.

87

Animal products such as meat, fish, milk and eggs contain small quantities.

As vitamin C is easily destroyed by heat, prolonged cooking of any food may destroy much of the vitamin C present.

Human requirements. Opinions regarding human requirements differ widely. It seems clear that as much as 75 mg/day is necessary if the body is to remain fully saturated with vitamin C. However, individuals appear to remain healthy on intakes as low as 10 mg/day. A recommendation of 25 mg for an adult, 30 mg for adolescents, 35 mg during pregnancy and 45 mg during lactation seems to be a reasonable compromise.

Scurvy and the other clinical manifestations of vitamin C deficiency are described on p. 111.

VITAMIN D

History. This vitamin is associated with the disease rickets and its adult counterpart osteomalacia. As vitamin D is produced in the human by the action of the sun on the skin, deficiency is not common in tropical Africa, although synthesis of vitamin D may possibly be reduced in darkly pigmented skin.

Although rickets was for many years suspected to be a nutritional deficiency disease, and in certain parts of the world cod-liver oil had been used in its treatment, it was not until 1919 that Sir Edward Mellanby, using puppies, demonstrated conclusively that the disease was indeed of nutritional origin, and that it responded to a vitamin present in cod-liver oil.

At first there was some confusion, as it was already known that cod-liver oil contained vitamin A, and it was only later that a second fat-soluble vitamin was isolated and called vitamin D.

Properties. A number of compounds, all sterols closely related to cholesterol, possess antirachitic properties. It was found that when ultraviolet light acted on certain sterols that did not have antirachitic properties, they became antirachitic. The two important activated sterols are vitamin D_2 (calciferol) and vitamin D_3 (cholecalciferol).

In human beings, when the skin is exposed to the ultraviolet rays of sunlight, a sterol compound is activated to form vitamin D, which is then available to the body. This has exactly the same function as vitamin D taken in the diet. The latter is only absorbed from the gut in the presence of bile.

The function of vitamin D in the body is to allow the proper absorption of calcium. Rickets and osteomalacia, though diseases in which calcium is deficient in certain tissues, are caused not by calcium deficiency in the diet but by a lack of vitamin D which would allow proper utilization of the calcium present in the diet.

Units. Vitamin D is expressed in international units (IU); 1 IU is equivalent to 0.025 μg vitamin D_3.

Dietary sources. Vitamin D occurs naturally only in the fat in certain animal products. Eggs, cheese, milk and butter are good sources in normal diets. Meat and fish contribute small quantities. Fish-liver oils are very rich. Cereals, vegetables and fruit contain no vitamin D.

Storage in the body. The body has a considerable capacity to store vitamin D in fatty tissue and in the liver. An adequate store is important in a pregnant woman, to avoid predisposition to rickets in the child.

Human requirements. It is not possible to define human dietary requirements, because the vitamin is obtained both by the action of sunlight on the skin and also by eating foods containing vitamin D. There is certainly no need for adults to have any vitamin D in their diets, provided they are adequately exposed to sunlight, and certainly many children in Africa survive in good health on a diet almost completely devoid of vitamin D. It has been shown that 400 IU of vitamin D in fish-liver oil will prevent the occurrence of rickets in infants or children not exposed to sunlight. This amount seems to be a safe allowance. Rickets and osteomalacia, two diseases resulting from a deficiency in vitamin D, are described on p. 106.

III. DISORDERS OF MALNUTRITION

A logical classification of nutritional deficiency diseases and states is difficult. The attempt to label the various nutritional deficiency diseases according to their supposed aetiology — a deficiency of one particular nutrient — gives an over-simplified picture. Many of the diseases have more than one causative factor, and it is seldom that a diet is grossly deficient in only one nutrient, while providing adequate quantities of all the others.

There are nutritional disorders of the skin, nervous system, eyes, and other organs and tissues that cannot be dealt with under one nutrient because more than one nutrient is involved. There are, however, certain specific syndromes and diseases that do follow a definite pattern and are easily described. There are other disorders clearly of nutritional origin that fit into no particular descriptive category. To complicate the issue further, there are signs and symptoms due to organisms, injury and non-nutritional and non-infective diseases that may be difficult to distinguish from malnutrition.

A multiple diagnosis is frequently necessary in Africa. That is to say, a patient often has more than one specific disease. It is especially common for persons suffering from malnutrition to have another illness, for poor nutrition may make a person more prone to infection or other diseases. Similarly the onset of a disease in a person who is on a borderline diet may tip the balance and cause the manifestations of malnutrition to appear almost concurrently with the new disease.

After a short discussion of starvation and obesity, a description will be given of the classical nutritional diseases beriberi, pellagra, xeroph-thalmia, rickets, osteomalacia, scurvy, goitre and — most important of all — protein-energy malnutrition (kwashiorkor and marasmus). The nutritional anaemias and neuropathies, and some of the lesser nutritional disorders will also be considered.

13. UNDERNUTRITION AND OVERNUTRITION

Starvation (undernutrition)

The classic scientific description of starvation is that of grossly under-nourished prisoners-of-war and refugees. Similar conditions have occurred in Africa following famines. Major famines due to poor rains have in recent years ravaged the people in the Sahelian countries of West Africa, and parts of Ethiopia.

In individual cases starvation may be due to serious disease of the intestinal tract, to an illness such as cancer, tuberculosis, to insanity, or occasionally to poverty and unemployment. In young children there are different causes for the common disease of nutritional marasmus (see p. 123).

There are many degrees of undernutrition, ranging from mild to fatal. A healthy man can tolerate the loss of about one quarter of his weight, but when he loses more than this he becomes ill, and his life may be threatened.

For example, an average African male weighing 55 kg (120 lb) may be forced to reduce his energy intake drastically during a famine year. Lacking food, he burns up body reserves. He loses fat, his muscles diminish in size, and he becomes thin. At the same time he has a natural inclination to reduce his energy output (see p. 56). He is less energetic, and rests and sleeps more. The energy expenditure of an average adult African male doing no exercise is about 1 300 Calories per day. If the food situation improves, for example with the new harvest, he is able to eat more food and hence increase his energy intake. His appetite also increases and he regains his weight without having done his body any real harm. Many people have gone for 10 days or more without any solid food at all (but with drinks of water or fluids). Under these conditions loss of weight occurs without permanent damage. If, however, the person in this example loses over 13.5 kg (30 lb) and continues on an energy-deficient diet, then definite signs and symptoms of starvation will develop.

Clinical features of starvation. In starvation the subject first becomes thin, his skin becomes dry and hangs loosely. The hair loses its lustre, the pulse slows and the blood pressure is reduced. Hormonal disturbances cause amenorrhoea in women and impotence in males.

Oedema, sometimes called famine oedema, is a frequent feature of severe undernutrition. The bedridden patient looks puffy, the ambulant person has swelling of the dependent parts of the body such as the feet and legs. Anaemia commonly develops, but is seldom severe. Diarrhoea is nearly always present. It may start early on in starvation or may be a terminal event.

Preschool-age children are often severely affected. They develop nutritional marasmus and sometimes kwashiorkor. This is often accompanied by intractable diarrhoea, which may, in the very weakened child, lead to prolapse of the rectum.

The starving person usually has psychological and mental disturbances. His personality may change, his ability to concentrate may be lost, but usually he remains rational.

Concurrent with these signs and symptoms there may be evidence of deficiencies of vitamins and other nutrients. In Africa the mouth lesions of riboflavin deficiency and tropical ulcers commonly occur; in prisoners-of-war in the Far East the "burning feet" syndrome (intense burning of the soles) was a marked feature, but almost any symptom of deficiency disease may arise, dependent in each case on the diet.

Treatment. The basis for treatment is to provide adequate food in a form that can be utilized by the individual and to treat any specific conditions in the manner appropriate to them.

An African suffering mild undernutrition, but showing few signs of starvation, will often cure himself simply by eating whatever food becomes available at the end of a famine.

In severe starvation, institutional treatment may be necessary. The patient may have a huge appetite, but his disturbed digestive tract can seldom cope with a large intake of varied rich foods. Milk, bland foods and limited roughage form the basis for successful treatment. Treatment of the young child is similar to that described for kwashiorkor and nutritional marasmus (see p. 119).

Obesity (overnutrition)

Obesity is now a major nutritional problem of the United States, some countries of Western Europe, and prosperous people everywhere. It is a paradox and possibly a censure of world morality that a significant part of the population of the world is greatly concerned with the problems of eating too much, while half the world's population suffers from undernutrition or deficiency states.

Although occurring among certain individuals or groups of people in Africa, obesity is not so widespread a problem as in Europe or North America and is therefore given only passing reference here.

Obesity is caused by the consumption of more food than the body needs. More energy is ingested in food than is expended in exercise, work, basal metabolism, etc. Obesity is only very rarely due to endocrine dysfunction, or what is commonly called "glandular trouble", and even then there is an excess of energy intake over output.

The main and most obvious features of obesity are increased weight and fatness. In affluent countries severe obesity may cause psychological upset because people do not like to be conspicuous or thought ugly, but the unhappiness this causes may lead to eating more rather than less. In fact anxiety and unhappiness may be the cause of the original obesity. In Africa it is sometimes considered that obesity adds prestige to an individual.

Severe obesity may lead to difficulty in moving about, to tiredness and to arthritis in weight-bearing joints. It definitely reduces the life expectancy of the individual. In hot humid climates, skin infections are common in the groins and other flexures of obese subjects. Diabetes mellitus, varicose veins, high blood pressure and arteriosclerosis (including that in the coronary arteries) are all more prevalent in overweight persons.

Recent evidence suggests that overfeeding of infants and young children may lead to the production of increased numbers of fat cells in the body and predispose the individual to obesity in adulthood.

Treatment. The only logical way to treat obesity is to reduce energy intake and increase its expenditure. The former can be lowered by reducing the size of servings at each meal; the latter can be raised by increasing the amount of exercise taken. However simple this may sound, the successful long-term maintenance of lowered weight is very difficult in obese persons.

A reducing diet should always aim to limit energy intake without leaving the individual short of essential nutrients. Most satisfactory will be a reduction in the amount of predominantly carbohydrate and fat-containing foods, without much reduction in foods rich in proteins, minerals and vitamins, e.g., lean meat, fish, legumes, fruit or vegetables. There is no prophylactic treatment that will of itself induce weight loss.

The use of amphetamines, thyroid extracts and other drugs in the treatment of obesity is in general to be condemned and at best should be only under the careful supervision of an experienced doctor. Similarly, most of the highly advertised rapid-reducing diets, some even promoted by physicians, have been found to be ineffective and sometimes dangerous.

14. BERIBERI

Incidence in Africa

This disease is certainly not common in Africa, whereas it is or has been extremely prevalent in much of Asia. Doctors in various parts of the African continent have from time to time reported cases, but relatively few of them have been scientifically investigated or authenticated. Beriberi has occurred in special circumstances, such as among African troops fed on a rice diet, in male Bantu alcoholics in South Africa, and among predominantly rice-eating people in Egypt and West Africa, including the Congo. Beriberi is due to a deficiency of B vitamins, especially thiamine, when the ratio of its intake to the number of calories obtained from carbohydrate is low. The disease occurs predominantly among rice eaters. This almost exclusive association of beriberi with a rice diet is difficult to explain when comparing the thiamine content of milled cereals because many of them, including highly milled wheat and maize, are also low in thiamine. There have been a few authenticated cases of beriberi in wheat eaters and the fact that there are not more is possibly because most wheat eaters in the world are living at an economic level where they can afford a more varied diet.

Beriberi became a scourge as the milling industry expanded throughout Asia, producing polished rice, deprived of its thiamine content, for poor people at a financial cost no more than that of home-pounded rice, but at a cost of many thousands of lives. The milling industry in Africa is perhaps only just now reaching the stage with maize that it did in Asia with rice during the last century. Highly milled white maize-meal is rapidly becoming popular in Africa. Some countries have banned its manufacture, others are contemplating legislation to enforce vitamin enrichment.

A number of medical authorities feel that maize presents no real problem. Yet highly milled maize-meal as sold in much of Africa contains only 0.05 mg thiamine/100 g, compared with 0.06 mg in highly milled polished rice in endemic beriberi areas of the Far East. In contrast, lightly milled or hand-pounded maize and rice contain about 0.3 and 0.25 mg respectively. In highly milled maize-meal, the level of riboflavin is similar to that of rice, and the nicotinic acid content is lower. Why then has beriberi not become a major problem? Most likely because highly refined maize is eaten mainly by the better-off people who include other foods in their diet, and its use is only just beginning to spread to poorer groups. Furthermore, since maize contains a different ratio of B vitamins the classical syndrome of true oriental beriberi will seldom if ever occur in persons on a maize diet. However, certain cardiac conditions occasionally encountered in Africa may be due to thiamine deficiency.

In Madagascar heart disease related to thiamine deficiency has been reported. There is certainly a great deal of evidence of riboflavin deficiency among Africans and recently a number of peculiar neuropathies have been described. It is therefore important for nutrition and health workers in Africa to be familiar with the different manifestations of beriberi, so that they can look out for them. It is equally important that they keep an open mind, and report other syndromes that may indicate specifically African manifestations of thiamine and B vitamin deficiencies.

The disease

There are various ways of dividing beriberi into its clinical types. Here it will be grouped into three forms: wet beriberi, dry beriberi, and infantile beriberi. These conditions have many different features and yet appear to be caused by the same dietary deficiencies and occur in the same endemic areas.

Early clinical features common to both wet and dry beriberi. Both wet and dry beriberi usually begin in a similar mild way. The person feels unwell, his legs become tired, heavy, and appear to have less power, with some swelling toward evening. There may be a little numbness and some feeling of pins and needles in the legs, as well as occasional palpitations. The person may continue with normal activities, often, however, reducing his movements at home or at work, but seldom reporting to a doctor. If examined, he would be found to have a little loss of motor power of the legs, perhaps some alteration in gait, and areas of mild anaesthesia, often over the shin. The condition would improve with either a better diet or with thiamine. If left untreated, the condition might continue for months or years, but may at any stage progress to either wet or dry beriberi.

No satisfactory explanation has been given as to why in one case it goes one way, and in a second case the other.

Wet beriberi. The patient does not usually appear either particularly thin or wasted. The main feature is pitting oedema, which is nearly always present in the legs, but may also be seen in the scrotum, face and trunk of the body. The patient usually complains of heart palpitations and chest pain. There is dysponea (breathlessness), a rapid, sometimes irregular, pulse and distended neck veins with visible pulsations. The heart is found to be enlarged. The urine, which tends to be diminished in volume, should always be tested for albumin, either in the hospital ward or even in a small dispensary. In beriberi, no albumin is present, and this is very important in helping the diagnosis in a case with oedema.

A patient with wet beriberi, even if he looks reasonably well, is in danger of very rapid deterioration of his condition with the development of sudden coldness of the skin, cyanosis, increased oedema, severe dyspnoea, acute circulatory failure and death.

Dry beriberi. The patient is thin, with weak, wasted muscles. Anaesthesia and pins and needles in feet and arms may increase, and gradually he has difficulty in walking, until he cannot walk at all. Before this stage is reached, he may develop a peculiar ataxic gait. Foot drop and wrist drop commonly occur. On examination, the main features are the wasting, anaesthetic patches (especially over the tibia), tenderness of the calves to pressure, and difficulty in rising from the squatting position. The disease is usually chronic, but at any stage improvement may occur if a better diet is consumed, or if treatment is begun. Otherwise, the patient becomes bedridden and frequently dies of chronic infections such as dysentery, tuberculosis or bedsores.

Infantile beriberi. This is the only serious deficiency disease that commonly occurs in otherwise normal infants under 6 month of age who are receiving adequate quantities of breast milk. It is due to inadequate thiamine in the milk of mothers who are deficient in this vitamin, though the mother often has no overt signs of beriberi.

It usually occurs in infants between their second and sixth months. In the acute form, the infant develops dyspnoea and cyanosis, and soon dies of cardiac failure. In the more chronic variety, the classical sign is aphonia, the child going through the motions of crying like a well-rehearsed mime, but without emitting any sound, or at most, the thinnest of whines. The infant becomes wasted and thin, vomiting and diarrhoea develop and, as the disease advances, the infant in fact becomes marasmic, due to deficiency of energy and nutrients. Oedema is occasionally seen and convulsions have been described in the terminal stages.

Diagnosis of wet, dry and infantile beriberi

Diagnosis is difficult when only the early manifestations are present. Evidence of a diet deficient in thiamine in an endemic area and of an improvement on a good diet both help to establish the diagnosis.

Wet beriberi must be distinguished from renal oedema and congestive cardiac failure. In both of these, there is albuminuria.

A diagnosis of dry beriberi may sometimes wrongly be made in a case of neuritic leprosy which has no obvious skin lesions. In neuritic leprosy the affected nerves, especially the ulnar and peroneal, are palpably thickened and cordlike, whereas in beriberi there is no enlargement. It is often extremely difficult to differentiate infective and toxic neuropathies from dry beriberi, but a full investigation into the patient's history is essential.

96

In acute infantile beriberi, the disease is so rapid in its course that diagnosis is very difficult. In the more chronic forms, loss of voice, among other signs, is characteristic of the disease. In both forms the mothers should be examined for signs of thiamine deficiency.

There are no really reliable laboratory tests for beriberi (none, at any rate, that are available in the average African hospital or dispensary). Electrocardiograph (ECG) examination does not give a definitive picture.

Treatment

Wet beriberi

1. Absolute bed rest.
2. Thiamine by injection, 10 to 20 mg daily; with improvement, stop injections and give 10 mg daily by mouth.
3. Full nutritious diet rich in foods known to contain thiamine (perhaps supplemented with the vitamin B complex) but low in carbohydrate.

Severe wet beriberi is a most gratifying disease to treat, for the response is in most cases rapid and dramatic.

Diuresis and lessening of dyspnoea is observed, and after a few days oedema disappears.

Dry beriberi

1. Rest in bed.
2. 10 mg thiamine daily by mouth.
3. Full nutritious diet rich in thiamine and supplemented with the vitamin B complex.
4. Physiotherapy or putting splints on joints, each case being treated on its merits.

Response to treatment tends to be rather slow, but deterioration of the condition is arrested.

Infantile beriberi

1. Injection of 5 mg thiamine when first seen.
2. 10 mg thiamine twice daily by mouth to the mother, if the child is being breast-fed.
3. If the mother is unavailable or the child is not being breast-fed, thiamine-rich products such as Marmite should be given to the child.

Prevention

1. Limitation or prevention of the sale of thiamine-deficient rice and other cereals by:

- Encouraging the consumption of lightly milled rice and other cereals;
- Legislation or other inducement to ensure that all rice put up for sale is either lightly milled, parboiled, or enriched;
- Legislation to ensure vitamin enrichment of cereals made deficient by milling.

2. Encouragement of the consumption of a varied diet containing adequate quantities of B vitamins, that is, if highly milled white rice is the staple diet, part of this should be replaced by a lightly milled cereal such as millet and supplemented with foods rich in thiamine.
3. Instruction in the most satisfactory ways of preparing and cooking foods in order to minimize thiamine loss.
4. Administration of thiamine either in natural food, yeast products, rice polishings or as tablets to certain vulnerable groups in the community.
5. Nutrition education to stress the cause of the disease and to indicate the foods that should be consumed and the ways of minimizing vitamin loss during food preparation.
6. Early diagnosis of cases of thiamine deficiency and appropriate measures of treatment and prevention.

15. PELLAGRA

This disease occurs in many countries of Africa, and especially where maize is the staple diet. It is uncommon in children. The previous assumption that it was a subtropical rather than a tropical disease and the belief that it occurred only in institutions or towns in the tropics are untrue. Many cases are seen among poor rural Africans living on subsistence farming very close to the equator. Admittedly the disease does not seem to occur among those eating millet or sorghum as their staple, and possibly the disease only reached Africa with the arrival of maize and cassava.

As mentioned under niacin (p. 82), a number of factors have at different times been suggested as the cause of pellagra. Each theory seemed, when first expounded, to oppose another. Three of the principal theories appear to have an element of truth. Pellagra was first thought to be due to a toxin in maize, then to a protein deficiency, and lastly to a lack of niacin in the diet.

It has now been found that maize contains more niacin than some other cereal foods, but it is believed that the niacin in maize is in a bound form. It is also now known that the human body can convert the amino acid tryptophan into niacin, and thus a high-protein diet, assuming the protein contains good quantities of tryptophan, will prevent pellagra. Despite all this, niacin is still the most important factor in pellagra, and any programme to prevent the disease should aim at providing adequate niacin in the diet. Similarly, all cases of pellagra should receive niacin therapeutically.

The disease

Persons suffering from pellagra usually appear poorly nourished. They are often rather weak and underweight. The disease is characterized by "the three Ds": dermatitis, diarrhoea and dementia (see Fig. 19).

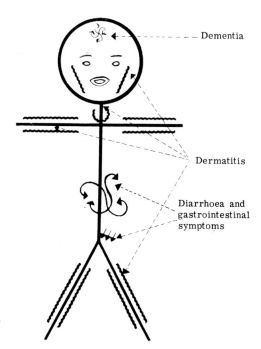

Dementia

Dermatitis

Diarrhoea and gastrointestinal symptoms

FIGURE 19. Characteristics of pellagra.

99

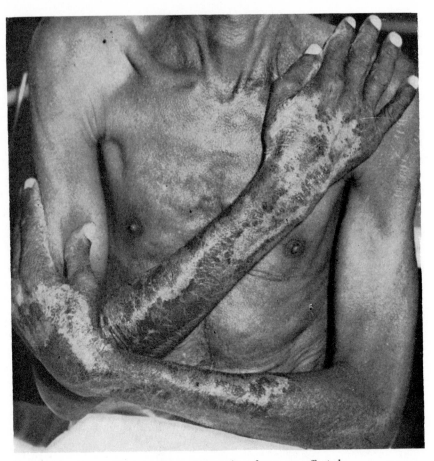

FIGURE 20. Dermatitis in pellagra. Exposed surfaces are affected.

Dermatitis. The disease is most often diagnosed from the appearance of the skin, which has characteristic lesions (see Fig. 20). This (pellagrous) dermatitis begins in the African with a deepening of the pigmentation. The hyperpigmented areas lose the oily sheen of healthy skin, and become dry, scaly and eventually cracked. There is usually a definite line of demarcation between these lesions and the healthy skin, and this line can be felt, for the affected area is rough to the touch. This condition may remain static, it may heal, or it may progress. If the latter, desquamation commonly occurs, or there may be cracking and fissuring, or occasionally the skin may become blistered. The blisters contain a colourless exudate. Areas that have shed a layer of skin are sometimes shiny, thin and rather depigmented. All these skin lesions are usually more

100

FIGURE 21. Casal's necklace in pellagra.

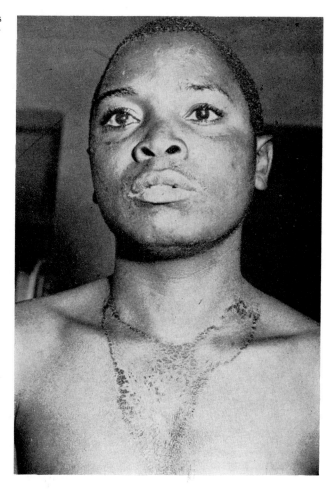

or less symmetrical. Most important of all they occur on areas of the skin exposed to sunlight, such as the face, the back of the hands, the neck, the forearms, and exposed portions of the leg.

In European cases, the skin lesion initially looks like the erythema of sunburn. Although Africans do not suffer from sunburn, the lesions of pellagra patients produce burning sensations and pain when exposed to the direct rays of the sun, just as sunburn does in a person with a pale skin. The lesions may also correspond with a hole in a frequently worn garment, the hole having allowed the sunlight to reach the skin. For example, the classic Casal's necklace (see Fig. 21) around the neck and upper chest is due to the sun playing on this part of the body in a subject wearing an open-necked shirt.

Diarrhoea. Bouts of abdominal pain, diarrhoea, and other digestive upsets are frequently associated with pellagra. The mouth and tongue may be sore. Angular stomatitis and cheilosis usually associated with riboflavin deficiency are frequently observed. The tongue and other parts of the mouth are often red, smooth and raw-looking. It is believed that similar changes are present in various other parts of the alimentary tract, and these may be the cause of abdominal discomfort and intestinal burning. Few if any of these symptoms and signs are specific to pellagra. But if they accompany skin changes or mental symptoms or respond to niacin, this supports a diagnosis of pellagra.

Dementia. Involvement of the nervous system manifests itself by extremely variable symptoms and signs. The commonest are irritability, loss of memory, anxiety and insomnia. These may lead to dementia, and it is not uncommon in African practice for these persons to be admitted to mental institutions. All cases of insanity in Africa should therefore be examined for other signs of pellagra.

Mild sensory and motor changes such as diminished sensation to gentle touch, some muscular weakness and tremor all occur. A wide variety of other signs has been described. Paralysis, however, is rare.

Diagnosis

The skin lesions are usually characteristic in appearance. The fact that the lesions are symmetrical and on surfaces of the body exposed to sunlight substantiates the diagnosis. The alimentary and nervous symptoms and signs are not often specific. The dietary history, the presence of skin changes, the appearance of the mouth, and, above all, the good response to niacin are characteristic. The urine is also low in niacin.

Treatment

1. Admission to hospital and rest in bed are desirable for serious cases. Milder cases may be treated as outpatients.
2. 50 mg of niacin (nicotinic acid, nicotinamide) should be given three times a day by mouth.
3. A diet containing at least 10 g/day of good protein (if possible, meat, fish, milk, or eggs; if not, groundnuts, beans, or other legumes), and with a high energy value (3 000-3 500 Calories/day) should be given. If intestinal symptoms are marked, the diet should be low in roughage.

4. Because there may also be a deficiency of other B vitamin components, a vitamin B complex preparation or a yeast product should be prescribed.
5. Sedation for a few days is recommended. Those with mental disturbances benefit greatly from any of a number of the more potent tranquillizers. This should be given orally unless the patient is uncooperative, when it can be given by injection.

Prevention

1. Discouragement of reliance on maize as the sole staple foodstuff, and encouragement of the consumption of other cereals in place of part of the maize.
2. Increased production and consumption of foods known to prevent pellagra, i.e., those rich in niacin, such as groundnuts, and those rich in tryptophan, such as eggs, milk, lean meat and fish.
3. Legislation or other inducement to ensure the enrichment of milled maize-meal with niacin and/or protein.
4. Prophylatic administration of niacin tablets in prisons and institutions in areas where pellagra is endemic.
5. Nutrition education to teach people what foods can prevent the disease.

16.   XEROPHTHALMIA AND KERATOMALACIA

Xerophthalmia, the general term used for vitamin A deficiency, has its most serious effects on the eyes when it causes softening of the cornea. This may lead to ulceration followed either by scarring or by secondary infection, panophthalmitis, and blindness (see Fig. 22). This very serious form of xerophtalmia is called keratomalacia. It occurs most commonly in young children, and is frequently associated with protein-energy malnutrition. The transport of vitamin A stored in the liver is dependent on a retinol-binding protein, which is nearly always very low in children with kwashiorkor.

Xerophthalmia is often precipitated by infectious diseases such as diarrhoea and measles.[1]

---

[1] It may also be induced by distribution of non-vitaminized dried skim milk in areas where the population suffers from protein-energy malnutrition (see FAO, 1977).

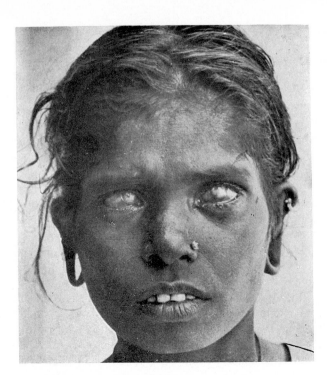

FIGURE 22. Kerato-
malacia

The disease

Night blindness frequently precedes other more serious changes in the
eye. In this condition the person has a reduced ability to see in dim light.
In a child this may not be noticed although sometimes the mother may
report that her son or daughter is clumsy in the dark or fails to recognize
people in a poorly lighted hut.

Another early sign of xerophthalmia is the presence of Bitot's spots
(described on p. 153). Advanced destructive lesions of xerophthalmia
may occur without Bitot's spots, which are therefore not a stage in the
disease process. However, Bitot's spots, when found in a survey, provide
good evidence that vitamin A deficiency is present in the community.

At later stages the conjunctiva dries out and loses its shiny lustre.
This is known as xerosis and is seen as dry patches on the conjunctiva.
This condition may then spread to the cornea, which also becomes dull
and loses much of its power to reflect. This pathological dryness of the
eye, from which the name xerophthalmia derives, deprives it of its epithelial
protection. Later still there is a gradual softening as a necrotic process
sets in. This leads to ulceration of the cornea. If untreated, the ulcer
perforates and secondary infection ensues. The patient may then become

seriously ill, often with a high fever and a grossly inflamed eye that is doomed to blindness. If treatment is started and if food rich in vitamin A is consumed before the stage of perforation, then the ulcer may heal, leaving perhaps a small opaque scar on the cornea. In some cases, vascularization of the cornea occurs before the stage of perforation.

A classification system for stages of xerophthalmia used by WHO (WHO, 1976) is given below.

Classification	Signs — primary
X1A	Conjunctival xerosis
X1B	Bitot's spot with conjunctival xerosis
X2	Corneal xerosis
X3A	Corneal ulceration with xerosis
X3B	Keratomalacia
	Signs — secondary
XN	Night blindness
XF	Xerophthalmia fundus
XS	Corneal scars

Treatment

Severe cases of keratomalacia are an emergency of some magnitude, and should be treated as such.

1. A water-miscible preparation of 55 mg of retinyl palmitate (100 000 IU vitamin A) should be given by intramuscular injection. This should be followed one day later by a similar dose in an oil preparation given orally. On leaving hospital, patients under 1 year should be given the same oral dose, and older ones twice the dose.
2. Tetracycline or other antibiotic eye ointment should be instilled into the eye every 4 hours.
3. If secondary infection is present, give 600 000 units of penicillin or some other antibiotic daily by intramuscular injection.
4. Supply a good mixed diet rich in vitamin A, carotene and protein.

Prevention

1. General measures should be introduced to reduce poverty and improve standards of living, including steps to assist the provision of an adequate diet, of better home and personal hygiene, and of better education in the community.

2. The greater production and consumption, especially by children, of foods containing good quantities of vitamin A or carotene, e.g., green leafy vegetables, certain fruits, red palm oil, dairy products and eggs. Horticultural activities designed to increase the production of local high-carotene fruits and vegetables.
3. Fortification of a suitable food (or food additive) with vitamin A; those that have been considered include cereal flours, salt, sugar, tea and monosodium glutamate.
4. Mass dosing of vulnerable children in a community with 110 mg of retinyl palmitate in oil (200 000 IU vitamin A) given orally every 4-6 months will protect young children from xerophthalmia. The vitamin A is stored in the liver.
5. Nutrition education, especially stressing the need to consume foods rich in carotene or vitamin A as part of a balanced diet. These can include wild leaves and fruits that are traditionally eaten in the area.
6. Cooperation with officials of the Ministry of Agriculture to ensure a coordinated policy. For instance, the nutrition or health worker can inform the agriculturist as to the extent of the problem and what foods will solve it. The agriculturist can decide which carotene- or vitamin A-rich foods are most suitable for local production.

17. RICKETS AND OSTEOMALACIA

RICKETS

Rickets results from a lack of calcium in the body, due not so much to a diet inadequate in calcium as to defective calcium absorption arising from a deficiency of vitamin D. The disease occurs in infants and young children. As mentioned earlier, vitamin D can be obtained either from animal foodstuffs in the diet, or it can be manufactured by the body if the skin is adequately exposed to sunlight.

Serious cases of rickets are uncommon in most tropical African countries, not because of animal foodstuffs consumed but because of the sunshine. It has been reported from persons living in dense shady forests (Guinea and the Ivory Coast), and it occurs in children who are confined to rooms or dark backyards of city homes (South Africa), and in infants who are overclothed (Yoruba, Nigeria) or who, for some other reason, do not have their skin adequately exposed to sunlight. Rickets is quite prevalent in Ethiopia. The only advanced case encountered by the author in Tanzania was the child of an Asian family practising strict purdah.

Rickets does frequently occur in the tropics but is much commoner in Asia and the Near East in the larger, more crowded cities with dark yards and narrow sunless streets; under social systems that preclude the appearance of women, and therefore young children, in public places; and where clothing habits may result in the child being either swaddled or attached to the mother in some way that leaves little skin exposed.

The diets of many African children after they are weaned tend to be very deficient in calcium, but a calcium deficiency alone has, surprisingly enough, never been proved to produce rickets.

The disease

In rickets, unlike most other deficiency diseases, the child often appears to be plump and well fed because the energy intake is usually adequate. This frequently misleads the mother into thinking all is well. The story has often been told of the rachitic child winning a baby show, because it appeared so fat and well nourished. The child, however, tends to be miserable, and closer examination will reveal the flabby toneless state of the muscles that causes a pot-belly. Another feature of the disease is the general impairment of normal development (see Fig. 23). A child is late reaching all the milestones in his early life. He is slow to learn to sit, slow to walk and slow to get teeth. Other generalized symptoms include gastrointestinal upsets and excessive sweating of the head.

However, the main signs of the disease and those on which the diagnosis of rickets is made are bone deformations. The first and main feature of this is a swelling at the growing ends (epiphyses) of the long bones. This may first be found at the wrist where the radius is affected. Another classic site is at the junctions of the ribs with their costal carti-lages, where swellings occur. This produces a beadlike appearance known as "rickety rosary". Swellings of the epiphysis of the tibia, fibula and femur may also be seen. In infants the anterior fontanelle closes late in rickets, and in older children a bossing of the frontal bone is found.

Once a child with rickets begins to stand, walk and become active, he develops new deformities due to the soft, weak character of the bones. The commonest of these is bowlegs, and, less frequently, knock-knees. More serious, however, are deformities of the spine. Changes in the pelvis, though often not visible, may lead to difficulty in childbirth in women who have had rickets.

For some unknown reason tetany has more frequently been reported in cases of rickets occurring in Africa than elsewhere. Tetany is due to

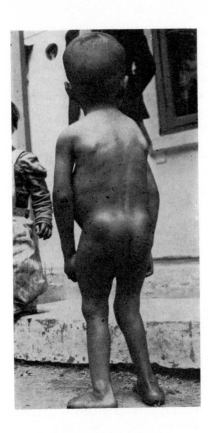

FIGURE 23. Child with a severe case of rickets.

a reduction in the level of serum calcium. It presents an unmistakable picture, with spasm in the hands, the thumb being drawn into the palm.

Rickets can be diagnosed by the characteristic X-ray changes in the bones. The level of serum alkaline phosphatase rises in cases of active rickets, whereas that of serum phosphorus drops well below normal levels.

Treatment

The basis of treatment is to provide vitamin D and calcium.

1. Vitamin D may be given as cod-liver oil. Three teaspoonfuls three times a day will supply about 3 000 IU, which is adequate. Synthetic calciferol can also be used. Calcium is best given as milk, at least half a litre a day. Cow's milk contains 120 mg calcium/100 ml.

2. Tablets containing vitamin D and calcium are available. One of these may be given twice a day to a child under 5 years of age, and three times a day to an older child.
3. Simultaneously with treatment, the mother should be educated regarding the value of sunshine. Rickets, unless severe, is not usually a fatal disease *per se*, although the child may be more prone to infectious disease.
4. Mild bone deformities tend to right themselves with treatment, but in more severe cases some degree of deformity may persist. One of the more serious results of such deformity is obstructed childbirth due to pelvic abnormalities. Sometimes this may mean that the woman must be delivered by caesarean section in hospital.

Prevention

1. Measures to ensure that all children get adequate amounts of sunlight. In temperate climates these include slum clearance; smoke abatement; the provision of parks, playgrounds, open yards and gardens; and regular outings for the young.
2. Adequate calcium and vitamin D in the diets of children (milk and milk products are especially valuable).
3. Regular clinic attendance of children so that early diagnosis of rickets can be made and curative measures taken.
4. Where item 1 above is not possible, vitamin D supplements such as cod-liver oil should be given to children.
5. Nutrition education regarding the needs for calcium and vitamin D and the methods by which adequate amounts of them can be obtained.

OSTEOMALACIA

Osteomalacia is the adult equivalent of rickets, being a deficiency disease associated with a lack of calcium in the bones. This is due usually to inadequate vitamin D in the body. It occurs more often in women than men. It is commonest in those women on a poor diet who have been depleted of calcium by years of pregnancies and lactation, who get little vitamin D in their diet, and who are mainly confined indoors. A lactating woman loses 30 mg of calcium in each 100 ml of milk, or as much as 93 grams of calcium per year, on the assumption that she produces 850 ml milk per day.

The disease

The patient usually walks with his or her feet rather widely separated and may appear to waddle. Deformities of the pelvis may be obvious. Tetany may occur. This may be seen as involuntary twitching of the muscles of the face or by carpopedal spasm (the hand goes into rigid spasm with the thumb pressed into the palm). Pain occurs in the bones, commonly the pelvis, lower back and legs. Tenderness may sometimes be elicited in the shins or in other bones. Spontaneous fractures may occur. Before the deformities are clinically detectable, diagnosis may be made by X-ray examination. This will show rarefaction or decalcification of bones all over the body. Osteomalacia should not be confused with osteoporosis, a disease of ageing, in which decalcification is also a feature.

Treatment

The treatment is similar to that for rickets.

1. A dose of 50 000 IU vitamin D should be given daily as cod-liver oil or in some other preparation.
2. Calcium should be provided either as milk or, if this is not available, in some medicinal form such as calcium lactate.
3. In women with deformed pelves, regular antenatal care is essential and, in some cases, caesarean section before term may be necessary.

Prevention

1. Adequate exposure of the body to sunlight (this may conflict with religious or social customs, e.g., those requiring women to be heavily covered or veiled, or those forbidding women to go out in public).
2. Ensure that a diet containing adequate quantities of calcium and vitamin D are consumed, especially by pregnant and lactating women.
3. Establishment of clinics or home-visiting to allow pregnant and lactating women to be examined, and, where necessary, for the issue of cod-liver oil or other vitamin D supplements. Advice should be given regarding the consumption of calcium-rich foods; sometimes medicinal calcium (e.g., calcium lactate) will have to be prescribed.
4. Nutrition education, including child-spacing.

18. SCURVY

Many African diets are rather low in vitamin C. Nevertheless, scurvy, the serious disease resulting from a severe deficiency of vitamin C, appears to be rare in Africa. It occurs in persons who have for some considerable time eaten a diet containing very little fresh food. Vitamin C is necessary for the formation and healthy upkeep of intercellular material (see p. 86). In scurvy the walls of the capillaries lack solidity and become fragile, leading to haemorrhages.

The disease

The following symptoms and signs may occur:

● Tiredness and weakness;
● Gums become swollen and bleed easily at the base of the teeth;
● Haemorrhages occur in the skin;
● Other haemorrhages occur, e.g., nosebleeds, blood in the urine or faeces, splinter haemorrhages below the fingernails, subperiosteal haemorrhages;
● Delayed healing of wounds;
● Anaemia.

A patient with scurvy and having some of the above symptoms, though not appearing very seriously ill, may suddenly die of cardiac failure.

Subclinical vitamin C deficiency may result in the slow healing of wounds or ulcers. Vitamin C (ascorbic acid) should be given to patients who may be deficient and who are to have a surgical operation.

Infantile scurvy (Barlow's disease). Scurvy occurs sometimes in infants, usually aged 2 to 12 months, who are being bottle-fed with inferior brands of processed milk. During the processing of the milk, the vitamin C is frequently destroyed by heat. Good brands of processed milk are fortified with vitamin C to prevent scurvy.

The first sign is usually painful limbs. The infant cries when the limbs are moved or even touched. The child usually lies with the legs bent at the knees and hips, widely separated from each other, and externally rotated. Bruising of the body may be seen, though this is difficult to detect in darkly pigmented African skin. Swellings, however, may be felt, especially in the legs. Haemorrhages may occur from any of the sites mentioned above, but bleeding does not take place from the gums unless there are teeth.

Diagnosis

The capillary fragility test used in diagnosis in pale-skinned people is less useful in Africans. Ascorbic acid estimations of the blood or white blood cells (leucocytes) may help since, if ascorbic acid is present, the disease is not scurvy. The use of X-rays assists the diagnosis of infantile scurvy.

Treatment

Because of the risk of sudden death, it is inadvisable to treat scurvy with only a vitamin C-rich diet. It is advisable rather to give 250 mg ascorbic acid by mouth four times a day, and to put the patient on a diet with plenty of fresh fruit and vegetables. It is only necessary to inject ascorbic acid if the patient is vomiting.

Prevention

1. Increased production and consumption of vitamin C-rich foods, such as fruit and vegetables.
2. Provision of vegetables, fruit and fruit juice to all members of the community, including and beginning with children in the fifth month of life.
3. Provision of vitamin C concentrates if for any reason items 1 or 2 above are not possible.
4. Improved horticulture, including the provision of village and household gardens, orchards and vegetable allotments in towns and school gardens.
5. Encouragement of the wide use of edible wild fruits (e.g., baobab fruit) and vegetables known to be rich in vitamin C.
6. Action to avoid and discourage the replacement of fresh vegetables, fruit and other foods by canned and preserved foodstuffs. Encourage the greater use of fresh fruit and juices in place of bottled products.
7. Nutrition education, which should include the reasons and need for eating fresh foods, and instruction in means of minimizing vitamin C loss in cooking and food preparation.

Although scurvy is rare in Africa as a disease, swelling and bleeding of the gums occur fairly frequently in certain regions. This, together with slow healing of wounds and ulcers, may be due to vitamin C deficiency.

19. PROTEIN-ENERGY MALNUTRITION

Protein-energy malnutrition (PEM), also known as protein-calorie malnutrition, is today the most serious nutritional problem in Africa and other developing areas. Its two main clinical forms are kwashiorkor and marasmus. In the former, the main deficiency is one of protein; in the latter energy (calories).[1]

There are, however, many intermediate cases that are difficult to fit into either category. Again many children are deficient in protein and energy, suffer growth failure, and are predisposed to kwashiorkor and marasmus, but do not show any obvious warning symptoms or signs other than growth retardation.

KWASHIORKOR

In the severe form of protein-energy malnutrition known as kwashiorkor, the diet may be sufficient to assuage hunger, but is usually grossly deficient in protein and also in energy. The diet is therefore nearly always mainly carbohydrate, as well as being too small in amount for the needs of the child. The condition is often associated with an infectious disease.

Kwashiorkor occurs most frequently in children between 1 and 3 years of age, after they have been taken off the breast. While they are getting good quantities of breast milk, they are usually getting enough protein of good nutritional quality, containing all the amino acids essential for health and growth.

The immediate cause for stopping breast-feeding is frequently the realization by the mother that she is pregnant again. She may often believe that her milk will now poison the child, who is therefore taken away from the breast. There are of course other reasons why mothers stop breast-feeding their babies early, including the need for some mothers to work or live away from home. The young child may then be put on a diet of gruel or *uji* of whatever is the staple food of the family. This may be maize, cassava, banana, millet, rice, sorghum, or sometimes wheat. The child is sometimes sent away to live with a relative, frequently a grandmother, in order to make the process of complete weaning easier.

A young African child up to this time has usually had an extremely close relationship with his mother. He has ridden on his mother's back

---

[1] The Joint FAO/WHO Expert Committee on Nutrition (FAO, 1976) states "There is widespread agreement that kwashiorkor usually results from consuming food deficient in protein relative to calories and that marasmus is the consequence of insufficient food."

when she went to draw water or to till the field, he has slept in the same bed, he has had access to the breast more or less on demand. The sudden removal from this intimacy is a severe psychological shock, which may cause the child to lose his appetite, and may therefore be a factor in causing kwashiorkor. In more than one tribal tongue, the term for kwashiorkor is the equivalent of "displaced person". The child has been displaced by the foetus in his mother.

Other diseases may sometimes play an important role in precipitating the onset of true kwashiorkor in an already poorly nourished child. Among the most important of these are gastrointestinal infections, which cause diarrhoea and may hinder proper absorption of nutrients. They may also result in vomiting, and thus loss of food. Intestinal worms and other parasitic infections may be important, as well as measles, whooping cough and other infectious diseases. Nearly all infectious diseases lead to an increased loss of nitrogen from the body. This can only be replaced by protein in the diet.

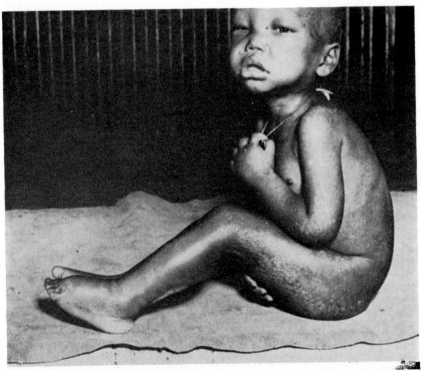

FIGURE 24. Kwashiorkor. This child shows oedema of the legs and face, dermatosis of the thigh, arm, and back. The oedema masks muscle wasting and growth failure.

114

The disease

Growth failure always occurs. If the child's precise age is known, he will be found to be shorter than normal and, except in cases of gross oedema, lighter in weight than normal (usually between 60 and 80 percent of standard). These signs may be obscured by oedema or ignorance of the child's age.

Wasting of muscles is also typical but may not be evident because of oedema.

Oedema causes swelling owing to the fluid in the tissues, and is always present. It usually starts with a slight swelling of the feet and often spreads up the legs (see Fig. 24). Later, the hands, scrotum and face may also swell (see Fig. 25). To diagnose the presence of oedema the medical attendant presses with his finger or thumb above the ankle. If

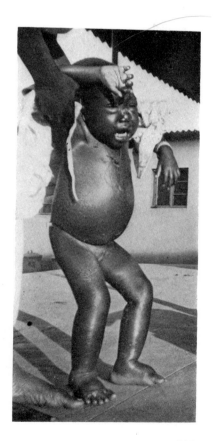

FIGURE 25. Oedema in kwashiorkor. This unhappy child has generalized swelling due to oedema. This masks muscle wasting and growth failure.

115

oedema is present the pit formed takes a few seconds to return to the level of the surrounding skin.

Mental changes are not invariably noticed. The child is usually apathetic about his surroundings and irritable when being moved or disturbed. He prefers to remain in one position and is nearly always miserable (see Fig. 26).

Hair changes. The hair of a normal African child is usually dark black, coarse in texture, and has a healthy sheen that reflects light. In kwashiorkor, the texture often changes, with the hair becoming silkier and losing its tight curl. At the same time it lacks lustre, is dull and lifeless, and may change colour to brown or reddish brown. Small tufts can sometimes be easily and almost painlessly plucked out. On examination under a microscope, plucked hair exhibits root changes and a narrower diameter than normal hair. The tensile strength of the hair is also reduced.

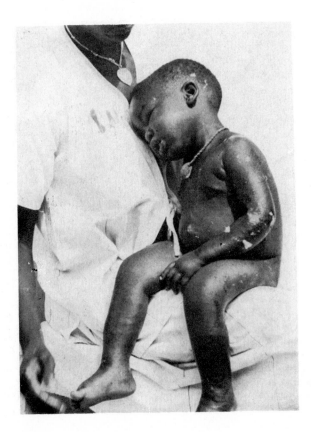

FIGURE 26. Kwashiorkor. Oedema, skin changes, and an ulcer near the elbow.

116

Skin changes. The skin, especially of the face, may be considerably lighter in colour than that of either parent. In some cases a dermatosis develops; this tends to occur first in areas of friction or of pressure, for excample, the groin, behind the knees and at the elbow. Darkly pigmented patches appear, which may peel off or desquamate, rather like old sun-baked, blistered paint. This observation has given rise to the term "flaky-paint dermatosis" (see Fig. 27). Underneath these flakes are atrophic depigmented areas that may resemble a healing burn. These areas may become secondarily infected. Skin cracks leading to ulceration may also occur.

Diarrhoea. Stools are frequently loose and contain undigested particles of food. Sometimes they are offensive, watery, or blood-stained.

Anaemia. Few cases do not have some degree of anaemia. This is due to lack of the protein required to synthesize blood cells. Anaemia may be complicated by iron deficiency, malaria, hookworm, etc.

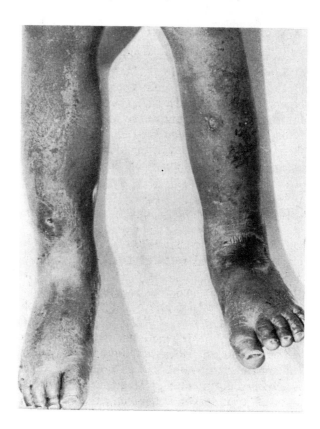

FIGURE 27. Flaky-paint dermatosis of kwashiorkor.

Hepatomegaly. The liver may be palpably enlarged. This is due to fatty infiltration of the liver, which is always found post-mortem in cases of kwashiorkor.

Moonface. The cheeks appear to be swollen either with fatty tissue or oedema fluid, giving the characteristic appearance known as "moonface". This condition occurs most often in children who have relatively little wasting and some oedema. The cause is unknown.

Signs of other deficiencies. In kwashiorkor, some subcutaneous fat is usually palpable. The amount of this fat gives an indication of the degree of energy deficiency. Mouth and lip changes characteristic of vitamin B deficiency are quite commonly found. Xerosis or xerophthalmia due to vitamin A deficiency is occasionally seen.

Findings in special laboratory tests. Serum proteins are reduced, the albumin content being more affected than the globulin. The serum amylase is reduced. Examination of duodenal juice reveals reduction in pancreatic enzymes.

Kwashiorkor is an extremely serious disease, and is a frequent cause of death in young children. Many mild cases occur that are not noticed by the parents, and therefore are never diagnosed. In these, recovery occurs if the child receives more protein and an adequate intake of energy. In severe cases with any of the above symptoms and signs, the outcome is likely to be fatal unless the child receives proper treatment. In all cases there is fatty infiltration of the liver but whether this results in any added risk of liver disease later is not known.

Differential diagnosis

Other possible long-term effects of kwashiorkor, such as permanent stunting of growth and retarded intellectual development, are discussed on page 128.
In trying to make a diagnosis, the conclusion that the child has kwashiorkor does not rule out other diseases also being present.

Nephrosis. If oedema is the main symptom of nephrosis, the disease may be confused with kwashiorkor. In nephrosis, however, the urine contains much albumin, and also casts and cells. In kwashiorkor, there is usually only a trace of albumin. If flaky-paint dermatosis or other signs of kwashiorkor are present, the diagnosis is established. Ascites is frequently seen in nephrosis, but only rarely in kwashiorkor. In Africa kwashiorkor is a much commoner cause of oedema than is nephrosis.

Severe hookworm anaemia. Oedema may result from this cause alone. In young children kwashiorkor is often also present. In pure hookworm anaemia, there would be no skin changes other than pallor. In all cases, the stools should be examined.

Chronic dysentery. In this disease oedema is not a feature.

Pellagra. This is rare in young children; the skin lesions are sometimes similar to those of kwashiorkor, but in pellagra they tend to be on areas exposed to sunlight (not the groin, etc.). There may frequently be diarrhoea and weight loss, but no oedema, hair changes, etc.

Treatment

1. *Hospitalization.* All severe cases should, if possible, be admitted to hospital with the mother and careful examination be made to reveal any infection. This will include a thorough clinical examination. A special search should be made for a respiratory infection such as pneumonia or tuberculosis. Stool, urine and blood examinations (for haemoglobin and malaria parasites) should be performed. The child should be weighed and measured.

Often hospital treatment is not possible. In that case the best possible medical treatment available at a health centre, dispensary or other medical facility is necessary.

2. *Diet.* Dried skim milk (DSM) powder often forms the basis of treatment.[1] DSM may most simply be reconstituted in hospital by adding 1 teaspoonful of DSM powder to 25 ml of boiled water and mixing thoroughly. The child should receive 150 ml of this mixture per kg body weight per day, given in six feeds at approximately 4-hour intervals. The milk mixture should be fed to the child with a feeding cup or a spoon but only if the child has sufficient appetite, is able to cooperate and is well enough. If not, the same mixture is best given through an intragastric tube. This tube should be made of polythene, be about 50 cm in length and have an internal diameter of 1 mm. It is passed through one nostril into the stomach. The protruding end should be secured to the cheek either with sticky tape or zinc oxide plaster. The tube can safely

---

[1] But see also the possible risk of using non-vitaminized DSM (footnote p. 103).

119

be left in position for 5 days. The milk mixture can best be given as a continuous drip, as for a transfusion. Alternatively the milk mixture can be administered intermittently using a large syringe and a needle that fits the tube. The milk mixture is then given in 4-hourly feeds. Before and after each feed 5 ml of warm, previously boiled water should be injected through the lumen of the tube to prevent blockage.

There are better mixtures than the plain DSM. They can all be administered, however, in exactly the same way. Most of these contain a vegetable oil (e.g., simsim, cottonseed), casein (pure milk protein, e.g., "Casilan-Glaxo"), DSM and sugar. The vegetable oil increases the energy content of the mixture, and appears to be better tolerated than the fat of full cream milk. Casein increases the cost of the mixture but, as it often serves to reduce the period in hospital, the money is well spent. A good and easily remembered formula for this sugar/casein/oil/milk (SCOM) mixture is: 1 part sugar, 1 part casein, 1 part oil and 1 part DSM, with water added to make 20 parts. A stock of the dry SCOM mixture can be stored for considerable periods of time in a sealed tin. To make a feeding, the desired quantity of the mixture is placed in a measuring jug and water added to the correct level. Stirring or, better still, whisking will ensure an even mixture. The amount to be given is the same as the pure DSM mixture previously mentioned, i.e., 150 ml of liquid mixture per kilogram body weight per day. This provides about 28 Calories, 1 g protein, and 12 mg potassium per 30 ml of made-up liquid feed.

EXAMPLES OF DIET TREATMENT:

A 5-kg child on plain DSM mixture

5 × 150 ml/day = 750 ml/day.
This is given in six feeds (i.e., one every 4 hours) = 125 ml/feed.
The DSM liquid mixture is made by adding 5 teaspoonfuls of DSM powder to 125 ml of water.

A 5-kg child on SCOM mixture

5 × 150 ml/day = 750 ml/day = 125 ml/feed.
The liquid SCOM mixture is made up by adding 5 teaspoonfuls of SCOM mixture to 125 ml of boiled water.

Both liquid mixtures may be administered by spoon, feeding cup or by intragastric tube.

3. *Medication.*

(*a*) Penicillin or some other antibiotic should be given to all serious cases of kwashiorkor, e.g., Benethamine Penicillin at 500 000 units, intra-muscular, daily for 5 days.

120

(*b*) In malarial areas, an antimalarial is desirable, e.g., half a tablet (125 mg) of chloroquine daily for 3 days, then half a tablet weekly. In severe cases and when vomiting is present, chloroquine should be given by injection.

(*c*) Potassium is desirable if dehydration exists, for it will serve to correct the electrolyte imbalance, e.g., 0.5 g potassium chloride (about 3 teaspoonfuls) in water, three times a day.

(*d*) If anaemia is very severe, it should be treated by blood transfusion and by intramuscular iron injection, using iron dextran (e.g., Imferon), 1 ml daily for about 5 days. In other cases ferrous sulphate mixture or tablets should be given.

(*e*) If a stool examination reveals the presence of hookworm, round-worm (*Ascaris*) or other intestinal parasites, then an appropriate anthelmintic drug should be given after the general condition of the child has improved.

(*f*) If vomiting persists, feeds should be given in smaller and more frequent amounts.

It is important to stress that every child with this disease must be treated on his or her merits as an individual. On the above regime, a serious case of kwashiorkor would usually begin to lose oedema during the first 3 to 7 days, with consequent loss in weight.

During this period, the diarrhoea should ease or cease, the child become more cheerful and alert, and skin lesions begin to clear.

When the diarrhoea has stopped, the oedema disappeared, and the appetite returned, it is desirable to stop tube-feeding, if this method has been used. The same SCOM or plain DSM mixture can be continued with a cup and spoon, or feeding bowl. A bottle and teat should not be used. If anaemia is still present, the child should now start a course of receiving iron by mouth, and half a tablet (125 mg) of chloroquine should be given weekly.

As recovery continues, usually during the second week in hospital, the patient gains weight. While continuing to supply milk, a mixed diet should gradually be introduced. This should aim at providing the necessary energy, protein, minerals, and vitamins for the child.

If the disease is not to recur, it is important that the mother participate in the feeding at this stage. She must be told what the child is getting and why. Her cooperation with and follow-up of this regime is much more likely if the hospital diet of the child is based mainly on products that she uses at home.

This is not feasible in every case in a large hospital, but the diet should at least be based on locally available foods. Thus in a maize-eating area, for example, the child would now receive a maize gruel with

121

DSM added. For an older child, crushed groundnuts can be added twice a day or, if custom prefers, the child can eat roasted groundnuts. A few teaspoonfuls of ripe papaya, mango, orange or other fruit can be given. At one or two meals per day, a small portion of the green vegetable and the beans, fish or meat that the mother eats can be fed to the child, after having been well chopped. If hen eggs are available and custom allows their consumption, the mother can watch the process of boiling or scrambling an egg for the child. Alternatively, a raw egg can be broken into some simmering gruel or *uji*. Protein-rich foods such as beans, peas, groundnuts, meat, sour milk or eggs are all important. Often protein-rich foods of animal origin are relatively expensive. They are not essential and a good mixture of cereals, legumes and vegetables serves just as well. If suitable vitamin-containing foods are not available, then a vitamin mixture should be given, because the plain DSM and SCOM mixtures are not rich in vitamins.

The above are just examples. If the diet of the area is based on bananas, these can be used instead of maize, in which case protein-rich supplements are even more important.

The child, after discharge from hospital, should attend the outpatient under-fives clinic regularly and should follow the regime for mild cases described below.

When mild or moderate cases of kwashiorkor are treated at home and not in the hospital, they should, if possible, be followed in the outpatient department or clinic. It is much better if such cases can attend separately (i.e., on some special afternoon or at a child-welfare clinic) rather than in the tumult of most outpatient sessions. It is desirable to have a relaxed atmosphere, and the medical attendant should have time to explain matters to the mother and see that she understands what is expected of her. It is useless just to thrust a bag of milk powder or other supplement at her.

Treatment as an outpatient should be based on the provision of a suitable dietary supplement but, in most cases, it is best that this supplement be given as part of the diet. The child should be weighed and the mother told how many teaspoonfuls to give per day, and shown a teaspoon. Many supplements are best provided by adding them to the usual food (such as gruel or *uji*) rather than as separate preparations. This is certainly so with powdered milk. The mother should be asked how many times a day she feeds the child. If he is fed only at family mealtimes, which is often only twice a day, then she should be told to feed him two extra times.

If facilities exist and it is feasible, the SCOM mixture can be used for outpatient treatment. This is best provided ready mixed in sealed polythene bags.

122

NUTRITIONAL MARASMUS

This is the other severe form of protein-energy malnutrition. Whereas in kwashiorkor the main deficiency is one of protein, in marasmus the main deficiency is one of food in general, and therefore also of energy. It may occur at any age up to about $3\frac{1}{2}$ years, but in contrast to kwashiorkor it is more common during the first year of life. It is in fact a form of starvation, and the possible underlying causes of it are numerous. For whatever reason, the child is getting neither adequate supplies of breast milk nor of any alternative food suitable for it.

Perhaps the most important precipitating causes of marasmus are infectious and parasitic diseases of childhood. These include measles, whooping cough, diarrhoea, malaria and other parasitic diseases. Chronic infections such as tuberculosis may also lead to marasmus. Other common causes of marasmus are premature birth, mental deficiency and digestive upsets (malabsorption, vomiting, etc.). The usual cause, however, is early cessation of breast-feeding. This may be due to death of the mother, failure of lactation, separation of the mother from the infant (because of family trouble, because she is a working mother, etc.), or the mother's desire to feed her baby from the bottle rather than the breast (she may be influenced by advertisements or alien cultures into believing that this is sophisticated or superior). Early cessation of breast-feeding does not, of course, necessarily lead to marasmus. However, a very high proportion of the population of tropical Africa does not have sufficient income to buy enough milk to feed a baby properly. The tendency therefore is to overdilute a purchased mixture. Similarly, few households have running water or the other items in their homes that facilitate the sterile preparation of bottles of milk for an infant. Even if a sufficient quantity of milk is being bought to provide adequate energy and protein, the child commonly develops a gastrointestinal infection, which starts the vicious circle leading to marasmus.

Another cause of marasmus found in certain parts of Africa is prolonged breast-feeding without the introduction of other foods, or enough of other foods. It is unusual for a mother to be able to produce sufficient breast milk to supply all the energy and other nutrients necessary for an infant over 6 months of age.

The disease

In all cases the child fails to grow properly. If the age is known, the weight will be found to be extremely low by normal standards (below 60 percent of the standard). In severe cases the loss of flesh is obvious:

the ribs are prominent, the belly, in contrast to the rest of the body, may be protuberant, the face has a characteristic simian (monkey-like) appearance and the limbs are very emaciated. The child is "skin and bones". An advanced case of the disease is unmistakable, and once seen is never forgotten (see Fig. 28).

The muscles are always extremely wasted. There is little if any subcutaneous fat left. The skin, which hangs in wrinkles, especially around the buttocks and things, when taken between forefinger and thumb will reveal the absence of the usual layer of adipose tissue.

Children with marasmus are quite often not disinterested like those with kwashiorkor. Instead the deep sunken eyes have a rather wide-awake appearance (see Fig. 29). Similarly, the child may be less miserable and less irritable.

The child usually has a good appetite. In fact, like any starving being, he may be ravenous. He often violently sucks his hands or clothing or anything else available. Sometimes he is heard making sucking noises.

Stools may be loose, but this is not a constant feature of the disease. Diarrhoea of an infective nature, as mentioned earlier, may commonly

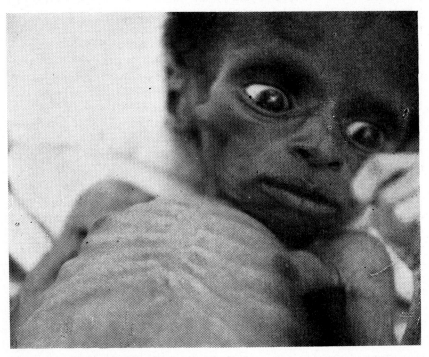

FIGURE 28. Severe nutritional marasmus.

have been a precipitating factor. Anaemia due to iron, protein and other deficiencies is usually present.

In contrast to kwashiorkor, there is no oedema and no flaky-paint dermatosis in marasmus. There may be pressure sores, but these are usually over bony prominences, not in areas of friction. Hair changes similar to those in kwashiorkor can occur. There is more frequently a change of texture than of colour. Dehydration, although not a feature of the disease itself, is a frequent accompaniment of the disease, and results from severe diarrhoea (and sometimes vomiting).

Treatment

Treatment for marasmus is similar to that for kwashiorkor. It is especially desirable, however, to see that adequate energy is supplied. It is very important to find the underlying cause. If this is an infective diarrhoea, dehydration may require special treatment with intravenous fluids or with intragastric tube feeding, but using a much more dilute

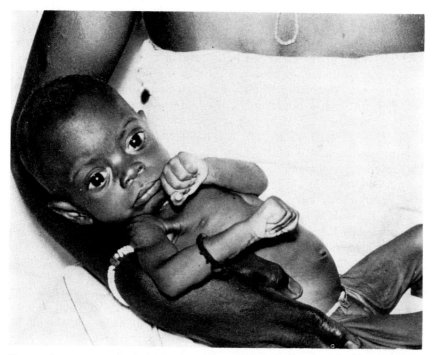

FIGURE 29. Marasmus, showing loss of subcutaneous tissue but bright, wide-awake eyes.

125

mixture than that recommended for kwashiorkor. If it is impossible to find a vein, then fluids can be given into the peritoneal cavity. Simultaneously sulphonamides or tetracycline should be given orally. Once the diarrhoea has been controlled, a nutritious high-energy diet is essential. The use of vegetable oil with DSM is even more important here than in kwashiorkor, as it will ensure a high energy intake.

Examination for tuberculosis is desirable. If there is any doubt, a tuberculin test should be performed, and if this is positive a chest X-ray should be taken.

Prognosis

The cause and the severity of the disease will determine the prognosis. A child with severe marasmus and lungs grossly damaged by tuberculous infection obviously has poor prospects. However, for a child with no other infection and mild marasmus, they are better. In any event response to treatment is likely to be slower than with kwashiorkor. It is often difficult to know what to do when the child is cured, especially if the child is under 1 year old. There may be no mother or she may be ill, and certainly she will have insufficient breast milk. Instruction and nutrition education of the person who will be responsible for the child are vital. If the child has been brought by the father, then some female relative should spend a few days in the hospital before the child is discharged. Instruction should be given in feeding with a spoon or cup, and not from a bottle unless the infant is under 3 months of age. The best procedure is usually to provide a thin gruel made from the local staple plus 2 teaspoonfuls of DSM (or some other protein-rich supplement) and 2 teaspoonfuls of oil per kilogram body weight per day. Instruction regarding other items in the diet must be given if the child is over 6 months old. The mother or guardian must attend the hospital or clinic at weekly intervals if she lives within, say, 10 kilometres, or at monthly intervals if further away. Supplies of a suitable supplement to last for slightly longer than this should be given at each visit. The child can be put on other foods, as mentioned in the discussion of treatment for mild kwashiorkor (p. 132), and of infant feeding in Chapter 36.

It is essential that the diet provide adequate energy and protein. Usually 120 Calories and 3 g of protein per kilogram of body weight per day are sufficient for long-term treatment. Thus a 10-kg child should receive about 1 200 Calories and 30 g of protein daily. It should be noted that a marasmic child, during the early part of recovery, may be capable of consuming and utilizing 150-200 Calories and 4-5 g of protein per kilogram body weight.

FIGURE 30. Characteristics of protein-energy malnutrition.

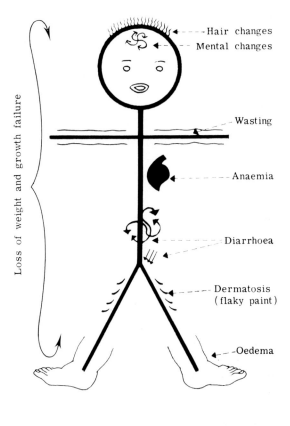

Loss of weight and growth failure

- - - -Hair changes
- - - Mental changes

Wasting

- - - - Anaemia

- - - - Diarrhoea

- - - - Dermatosis (flaky paint)

- -Oedema

INTERMEDIATE CASES

It is emphasized that kwashiorkor and nutritional marasmus are forms of protein-energy malnutrition. Kwashiorkor is the syndrome where the main deficiency is protein, and marasmus where it is one of food and energy (see Fig. 30). Cases with intermediate characteristics or that do not fit easily into either extreme category are not uncommon (often termed marasmic-kwashiorkor). This need not worry the medical attendant unduly, for the treatment is almost the same, and each patient should in any case be treated as an individual according to the clinical and other findings.

127

Comparison of the features of kwashiorkor and marasmus

Feature	Kwashiorkor	Marasmus
Growth failure	Present	Present
Wasting	Present	Present, marked
Oedema	Present (sometimes mild)	Absent
Hair changes	Common	Less common
Mental changes	Very common	Uncommon
Dermatosis, flaky-paint	Common	Does not occur
Appetite	Poor	Good
Anaemia	Severe (sometimes)	Present, less severe
Subcutaneous fat	Reduced but present	Absent
Face	May be oedematous	Drawn in, monkey-like

PROTEIN-ENERGY MALNUTRITION IN ADULTS

Though the term "adult kwashiorkor" has been used in some publications, it is probably better to reserve the word kwashiorkor for the disease in children, in whom it is very much more common and who often have certain features, such as flaky-paint dermatosis, that do not seem to occur in adults.

There is little doubt that a disorder does occur in adults due mainly to energy deficiency, and more commonly occurring in communities suffering from chronic protein-deficiency. The patient is markedly underweight for his height (unless grossly oedematous), the muscles are wasted and there is reduced subcutaneous fat. Mental changes are common, with the patient usually disinterested and appearing to be in a dream world. It is difficult to attract his attention and equally hard to keep it. Appetite is reduced, and the patient is very weak.

Some degree of oedema is nearly always present, and this may mask the weight loss, wasting and lack of subcutaneous fat. Oedema is commonest in the legs (see Fig. 31) and in male patients also in the scrotum, but any part of the body may be affected. The face is often puffy. This has been termed "famine oedema" because it occurs where there is starvation due to famine or other causes.

Frequent, loose, offensive stools may be passed. The abdomen is often slightly distended and, when palpated, the organs can be very easily felt through the thin abdominal wall. During palpation, there is nearly always a gurgling noise from the abdomen, and peristaltic movements can often be detected with the fingertips. It is not uncommon for these

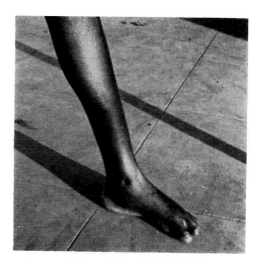

FIGURE 31. Oedema in the leg of an adult with protein-energy malnutrition. Note the pit near the ankle, made after applying pressure there.

patients to regard their physical state as emanating entirely from abdominal upset. For this reason, strong purgatives, either proprietary or herbal, or sometimes peppery enemas, which may have often greatly aggravated the condition, are often used by these patients before they reach hospital.

The hair frequently shows changes. There are more often changes of texture than of colour, though reddish brown hair is sometimes seen. The hair is much softer and silkier than normal, less curly and loses its reflective power and sheen. It may be a dull black rather than a shiny black (similar to black shoes when the polish is put on, but before they have been shined). Hair may be scantier than normal.

The skin is often dry and scaly, and may have a crazy-pavement appearance, especially over the tibia. The skin tends to desquamate, but unlike the dermatosis of classical kwashiorkor in children, it is not darkly pigmented, and when dry patches separate, there is not the pale pink, healed-burn appearance.

Swelling of both parotids is frequent. On palpation the glands are firm and rubbery. Anaemia is nearly always present and may be severe. The blood pressure is low. There is usually only a trace of albumin in the urine.

Although the above symptoms and signs are thought to be part of the disease, it is very difficult to separate them from many other symptoms frequently seen in these cases. These other symptoms are believed to be due to other disease processes that may be precipitating factors or just happen to be present. These may include angular stomatitis, soreness and redness of the tongue due probably to riboflavin deficiency, blood-stained stools or severe diarrhoea due to bacillary (or sometimes amoebic) dysen-

129

tery, tropical ulcers (in areas where these are common), heavy loads of hookworms and other intestinal parasites, malarial infection and spleno-megaly due to some of the above causes.

Treatment

Treatment for adult protein-energy malnutrition is on exactly the same lines as for protein-energy malnutrition in children, but a mixed diet high in protein and energy, as prescribed for children recovering from kwashior-kor or marasmus, can be introduced earlier. Care must be taken with the introduction of beans, which, although they are desirable because of their high protein content and availability, may be indigestible and increase flatulence. Tube feeding is rarely necessary. Particular care must be taken to treat allied infections. In severe anaemia, blood trans-fusion may cause rapid all-round improvement and shorten the stay in hospital.

Diferential diagnosis

Anaemia. Severe anaemia may also cause oedema. In PEM in adults, there is less dyspnoea and usually no cardiomegaly. Other features such as hair changes and parotid swelling are common in adult PEM but not in anaemia.

However, as lack of dietary protein appears to be a cause of anaemia, the two conditions are closely related.

MILD OR MODERATE PEM

The doctor finds it quite easy to diagnose both kwashiorkor and nutri-tional marasmus. These however are the extreme cases of protein-energy malnutrition, which may require hospital treatment and where the outlook for the child may be grave. Much commoner than these severe forms of PEM are what have been termed mild or moderate PEM.

Children with mild or moderate PEM do not have the gross oedema of kwashiorkor nor the emaciated appearance of nutritional marasmus. But they do have evidence of malnutrition and they are at special risk of developing the more severe forms of PEM, or of succumbing to an infectious disease. In most communities in Africa fewer than 5 percent (and frequently only 1 percent) of children at any one time have kwash-

130

iorkor or nutritional marasmus. But in these same communities usually at least 30 percent and sometimes as many as 75 percent of children have mild or moderate PEM.

The main feature of mild and moderate PEM is a failure to grow and develop optimally. Anthropometric measurements as described in Chapter 5 are used in determining these conditions. The commonest measurements, and the most useful, are weights and heights. If weights and ages of children are known in a community then the children can be classified nutritionally.

Bailey (WHO, 1975) has summarized the three main systems of classification according to body weight as follows:

Degree of malnutrition	Weight for age		Weight for height
	WHO method [1]	Gomez method [2]	Harvard standards [3]
	(Percentage of standard)		
Mild-moderate PEM	60-79	75-89 (Grade I)	80-89
		60-74 (Grade II)	
Severe PEM	Below 60	Below 60 (Grade III)	Below 80

[1] WHO, 1966 — [2] Gomez, 1956 — [3] See Appendix 2.

Although weight for age is a simple and useful means of classifying malnutrition, it fails to distinguish children who are currently malnourished from those who may at the time of examination be on an adequate diet, but who are underweight because of past chronic malnutrition.

If age, weight and height are known, then three different categories of malnourished children can be defined. These three groups include only children who have a low body weight in terms of standard weight for age. In addition to these three groups of malnourished children there would also be children whose weight and height were in the normal range and others who were obese or overweight. These would be classified separately as normal or overweight.

The three categories or types of malnutrition can be defined as follows:

Acute current short-duration malnutrition. This category includes children with normal height for age, low weight for age, and low weight

131

for height. Because height is normal but the weight is low, the child shows evidence of a recent short-duration deficiency of protein or energy.

Past chronic malnutrition. This category includes children with low weight for age, low height for age, but normal weight for height. The child shows evidence of a currently adequate intake of energy, but has the characteristic features of past long-duration malnutrition. Children who have recovered from this condition and nutritional dwarfs fit into this category.

Acute or chronic current long-duration malnutrition. This category includes children with low weight for age, low height for age, and low weight for height. The child shows evidence of both a past and present deficiency of energy or protein.

Just as the degree of malnutrition can be graded into three categories, so three levels of treatment and prevention might be considered.

The most serious cases of kwashiorkor and nutritional marasmus should be treated in hospital as already described. Wherever possible, hospital treatment should include nutrition and health education for the mother and child.

Some countries have established nutrition rehabilitation centres or mothercraft centres for the treatment, rehabilitation and prevention of PEM. These may form the second level of treatment.

The third level consists of several types of clinics variously called under-fives clinics, well-baby or health clinics, or childrens' outpatient clinics. Moderate or mild cases are suitably dealt with in these and also in the rehabilitation centres.

Nutrition rehabilitation centres and health clinics

Nutrition rehabilitation centres. Nutrition rehabilitation centres (NRCs) have been established in many countries in the last 10 to 15 years. The concept of these centres was originally propounded in 1955. They provide either sleeping accommodation for children or facilities similar to day nurseries or kindergartens, where malnourished children are either kept overnight or which they attend for a few hours each day. The objective is to educate the mothers through the nutritional rehabilitation of their children. The centres established in Asia, Africa, Latin America and the Caribbean often differ in the manner in which they function, but most have a common objective. An NRC differs from a day-care centre in several important respects:

The selection of children attending the NRC is based mainly on nutritional criteria, whereas day-care centres use social, educational, economic or other criteria for selecting their children.

132

The duration of attendance is usually based on the length of time necessary to rehabilitate the child, and is therefore limited.

Nutrition education of the mother is an important feature of the NRC.

The NRC caters for three groups: severely malnourished children after discharge from hospital during their important period of recuperation, moderately malnourished cases from the community, and less severely malnourished cases failing to make adequate progress following treatment as outpatients or at clinics.

In this graded system of treatment, children discharged from an NRC continue to attend some outpatient facility or clinic. In certain cases the NRC provides such a service at the centre.

The NRC has always been envisaged as providing important nutrition education. Another desirable feature is that it should be economical to run, and provide services at a fraction of the cost of hospitalization. An NRC could be an ordinary village house, staffed with one or two bright village women who have received some practical training in nutrition and child feeding. A typical NRC accommodates about 30 children who receive three or more good meals a day, and who attend 5 to 6 days per week for 8 to 10 hours per day for a period of 3 to 5 months. Mothers of children attending the centre are required to provide 1 day of work per week to assist with the running of the centre. The participation of mothers not only reduces the necessary staff but is especially important in providing an active learning experience. It may be used as such to teach improved child-feeding practices using local foods, and to instruct the mothers in other aspects of health and hygiene.

An NRC can play an important role in improving nutrition. However, the average centre — taking 30 children, each for 3 months — will provide services for only about 120 children per year. Very few countries can provide enough centres for all children with moderate malnutrition. If they are to have a real impact on nutritional problems in a country, they must be effective in nutrition education and also as demonstration and teaching centres.

Health clinics. Health clinics have been in existence in various countries for many years, and some have played an important role in reducing the incidence of certain deficiency diseases. In industrialized countries, rickets used to be very prevalent and a major cause of child mortality; the establishment of child clinics where cod-liver oil was dispensed and where attention to child health was provided was one of several factors responsible for its control. The term "under-fives clinics" is relatively new, and was coined by Dr David Morley in Nigeria.

The objective of these health clinics is to bring together the curative and preventive components of child-health care. There are advantages in separating these important activities aimed at children from the often overloaded outpatient services of hospitals.

There is no universal rule to indicate what services such a clinic should provide but, if at all possible, the clinic should be linked with some more sophisticated health unit; this may often be a hospital. This relationship may be close, as for example when a clinic is run as part of a general or children's hospital; or it may be remote and involve simple, occasional supervision from a hospital in the region or district. If the clinic is remote, a well-organized referral system and a means of transporting patients to hospital should be features of it. The professional staff in charge of these clinics can range from well-trained paediatricians to auxiliaries with a little special training in child health and nutrition.

The clinics should provide curative services at least for minor illnesses such as certain skin conditions, respiratory infections, parasitic diseases, diarrhoea including mild dehydration, and other common diseases.

Preventive medicine at the clinics should include at least two major components, namely immunization and nutrition services.

Immunizations should be available, preferably free, and parents should be encouraged to use this service for their children. In most countries the young child would receive: vaccination against smallpox; triple antigen (DPT) against diphtheria, pertussis (whooping cough) and tetanus; immunization against tuberculosis using BCG, against poliomyelitis using oral vaccine and against measles using live attenuated virus vaccine. In certain areas vaccination against other diseases such as cholera may be warranted. Some clinics may provide prophylaxis against malaria.

Nutrition activities are basically of two kinds: distribution of dietary supplements for malnourished children, and attention to growth and development of the child.

Supplements are designed to complement and add to the foods available at home for young malnourished children of poor families. The most widely used supplements have been protein-rich foods. Up to a few years ago these were mainly based on dried skim milk (DSM).

When DSM happens not to be available, a wide variety of protein-rich foods, many of them based on defatted soybean or other legumes, can be used. Currently food-aid programmes are providing CSM (corn/soybean/milk mixture), CSB (corn/soybean blend) and other blended foods for use in child-feeding programmes.

It has recently been realized that growth deficits in children, and mild or moderate malnutrition, are almost always due to a low total food intake and an energy deficiency, and are not often due solely to protein deficiency. Therefore a supplement providing a concentrated source of energy balanced with other nutrients, including protein, will be most frequently needed (see Chapter 36).

Attention to good growth and health development is perhaps the most important nutrition activity of health clinics. On each visit, every child should be carefully weighed and measured. Accurate scales, calibrated frequently, and good, simple equipment for measuring length or height are essential.

Recording the weight (and height) of children may serve three important purposes. It may help to detect children at high risk of developing PEM; it may be an important tool in assessing the effects of treatment; and most importantly, it can be used to follow the growth of the individual child. "Maintaining an adequate rate of growth" has replaced "prevention of malnutrition" as the goal toward which clinics should direct their work.

Experience has shown that the clinical syndromes of kwashiorkor and marasmus are usually preceded by months and sometimes years of failure to gain weight. The common exception to this is when a child develops kwashiorkor suddenly after an illness such as measles, whooping cough, or diarrhoea.

At health clinics, maintaining an adequate rate of growth has become a positive objective for both the staff and the mothers. A child who has failed to gain weight for several months is given special attention. In these clinics the mother is provided with a temporary supply of a food supplement, with instructions on improving the child's diet. The nurse uses the trend in the weight curve to assess the effectiveness of food supplements and of education in nutrition. If in spite of these measures failure to gain weight is persistent, the child is referred to a physician who examines him and where necessary undertakes laboratory and other procedures.

Many countries in Africa and elsewhere are using a growth chart, which the mother keeps. This chart, developed by Dr David Morley in Nigeria, and revised by WHO (WHO, 1978), includes: a calendar, for recording when the child was first seen, its age, recent and past medical history, state of nutrition, and inoculations received; and curves showing standard upper and lower limits of weight for age. Figure 32 shows a version of this chart adapted for monitoring PEM.

The calendar system has several advantages over many other methods of age-charting that record the age of the child in months. Monthly recording becomes increasingly difficult after the child is over 1 year old, since it requires a calculation (years $\times$ 12 + months) at each visit. This may lead to errors and be a deterrent to graphing weight, especially in a busy clinic.

On the Morley chart, entries are made of important incidents such as cessation of breast-feeding, birth of a sibling or major diseases at

FIGURE 32. Child's growth chart.

Date of visit			Weight	Arm circumference		
Day	Month	Year	kg	G	Y	R

corresponding points on the growth curve. With this chart the health worker can grasp the important facts of a child's medical history in a few seconds.

The chart, which should be colourful and durable, is usually supplied to the mother in a tough open-ended plastic envelope. It is considered to be her property and not that of the clinic. Experience in several centres has shown that few get lost, probably fewer than the number of records mislaid in the average small hospital's card-filing system. Indications for special care are written in a prominent position on the chart.

The following especially important factors have been noted as being commonly associated with low-weight children:

- Maternal weight below 43.5 kg;
- Birth order greater than seven;
- Death of either parent or a broken marriage;
- Deaths of more than four siblings, especially those occurring between 1 and 12 months of age;
- Birth weight below 2.4 kg;

136

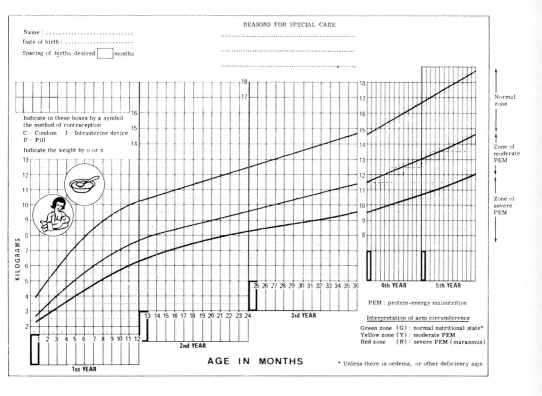

- Multiple births;
- Failure to gain 0.5 kg a month during the first 3 months of life, or 0.25 kg a month during the second 3 months;
- Breast infections in the mother and difficulties in breast-feeding, particularly those secondary to psychiatric illness in the mother;
- Occurrence of measles, whooping cough, and severe or repeated diarrhoea in the early months of life.

There is a considerable difference of opinion as to what weight standards should be used in developing countries. On Morley's chart an upper line is drawn to represent a satisfactory weight for a healthy, well-fed child at each age. A lower line indicates the tenth centile or some other arbitrary "standard", to indicate a level that the child should be above. The standard used is probably relatively unimportant. Of more significance than the position of the child's weight curve in relation to the "standard" is the relation of each weighing of the child to his previous weighings. The important point for the medical worker to watch is whether the child is following a path approximately parallel to the channel.

137

A number of biochemical tests and physical parameters that may help to identify a child in danger of developing PEM are currently under investigation. It must be realized, however, that for many years to come most children at clinics in developing countries will have to be seen by auxiliary personnel and not physicians, and their nutritional status will have to be determined by simple anthropometric means and not by biochemical tests (see page 25).

Clinic staff should spend as much time as possible providing *nutrition and health information*, either in groups or with individuals. Much has been written about the means of communicating nutrition and health facts to those with little education. Important points of nutrition teaching by clinic staff would be: to stress the value of breast-feeding; to emphasize the control of family size and spacing of children; and to pay attention to nutritional and health problems specific to the particular area.

The importance of operating a health clinic in conjunction with other health services cannot be overemphasized. The clinic itself or its facilities may also be used for antenatal clinics, which always need to be available for mothers to attend with their children and for family planning activities. The clinics themselves should in general be an important and integral part of the maternal and child-health services of the area.

Prevention

Preventive measures should aim at ensuring that all members of the community, especially young children and pregnant and lactating mothers, receive adequate quantities of energy, protein and other nutrients as part of a balanced diet. Preventive measures should also be directed at reducing the incidence of gastrointestinal infections (especially diarrhoea) as well as other diseases related to malnutrition. Thus, most measures related to improving the diet or the health of the community directly or indirectly assist in the prevention of protein-energy malnutrition. The most important practical measures to be taken will vary from area to area, but they should include the following:

1. Teaching mothers good weaning practices, i.e., encouraging breast-feeding to continue for as long as possible; at about 5 months of age to begin mixed feeding while continuing breast-feeding (the semi-solid foods introduced should include good quantities of protein-rich foods); after breast-feeding has ceased, the diet must contain adequate energy and good quantities of protein-rich foods. If for some reason breast-feeding is not possible in a child under 5 months of age, then some form of milk in adequate quantities is highly desirable.

2. Increasing production of all animal and vegetable foods rich in protein and ensuring their optimum use.

3. Providing protein supplements such as dried skim milk, and beans, at maternal and child-health clinics, and instructing mothers regarding their proper use.

4. Demonstrating the preparation and use of protein-rich foods and dishes for toddlers and young children (see p. 23).

5. Teaching people that it is vitally important to supplement predominantly carbohydrate staples liberally with protein-rich foods. This is very important when diets based on bananas and starchy roots such as cassava are the main food for toddlers.

6. Stressing the special dietary needs of pregnant and lactating mothers, and children, and in this context ensuring a fair distribution of food in the family.

7. Preventing gastrointestinal diseases, especially diarrhoea, in young children.

8. Ensuring proper treatment and, where possibile, the prevention of infectious, parasitic and other diseases.

9. Assessing the prevalence of protein-energy malnutrition by surveys, and ascertaining the relative incidence of kwashiorkor and marasmus. The staff at all medical units should be made fully aware of all details of diagnosis, treatment and prevention.

10. Correcting any harmful nutritional customs.

11. Promoting nutrition and health education.

12. Improving education, medical facilities, food supplies and the economy of the community. A better standard of living can assist disease prevention.

13. Encouraging the spacing of pregnancies.

14. Encouraging simple food storage, processing and marketing measures.

20. ENDEMIC GOITRE

Any swelling of the thyroid gland is called a goitre. This gland is centrally situated in the lower front part of the neck. In areas where only sporadic goitre occurs, it may be due to any of a number of causes not related to the individual's diet, and not therefore relevant to this book. However, where it is common or endemic in a community or district, the origin is usually nutritional.

Endemic goitre is commonly benign and does not often cause the symptoms and signs associated either with excessive or diminished secretion of thyroxine, the hormone of the thyroid gland. These conditions are described in textbooks of medicine.

Where goitre is endemic, frequently large numbers of people have an enlargement of the thyroid gland and some have enormous unsightly swellings of the neck. The condition is usually more common in females, especially at puberty and during pregnancy. The enlarged gland may be smooth (a colloid goitre) or it may be lumpy (an adenomatous, or nodular goitre).

The commonest cause of endemic goitre is a lack of iodine in the diet. The amount of iodine present in the soil varies from place to place, and this affects the quantity in both the food grown and the water supply in a given area. Seafoods are rich sources of iodine. Endemic goitre is generally more prevalent in plateau or mountain areas some distance from the sea, though there are exceptions.

Certain foods, if eaten in considerable quantities, predispose a person to goitre even if he is consuming normal quantities of iodine. These so-called goitrogenic agents occur in certain varieties of cabbage, kale, turnips and some other vegetable foods.

Water containing much calcium and other minerals, derived usually from the soil and said to be hard water, appears to inhibit the proper utilization of iodine in the diet. This may be a related factor in the aetiology of endemic goitre.

Incidence

Relatively few surveys have been carried out to ascertain the prevalence of goitre in the different districts of East Africa, but it is thought to be common in some areas. During a survey in the Ukinga Highlands of the Njombe District in Tanzania, the author examined 3 242 people and found that 2 448 had goitre, an incidence of about 75 percent (see Fig. 33).

When investigating goitre incidence it is advisable to examine the thyroid gland, both visually and by palpation, in order to estimate the degree of enlargement. A useful classification of goitre size into groups is that suggested by WHO (WHO, 1960), which is summarized below.

Group	Symptoms
0	Persons without goitre and persons with a thyroid less than five times enlarged. (Each lobe of a normal thyroid gland is about the size of the thumb-nail of the subject being examined.)
1	Persons with palpable thyroids more than five

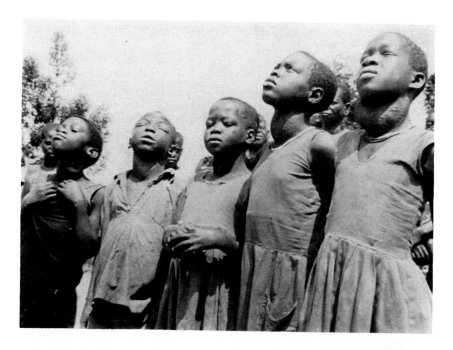

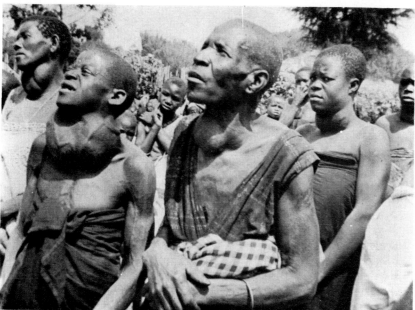

FIGURE 33. Goitre in the Ukinga Highlands, Tanzania. *Above:* in children. *Below:* In adults.

141

times enlarged, but not easily visible with the head in normal position.

2   Persons with goitres easily visible with the head in normal position, but which are smaller than those in Group 3.

3   Persons with large goitres easily recognizable at a considerable distance and which may be disfiguring.

Treatment

Iodine therapy. Iodine given by mouth will cure many, and reduce the size of some, goitres, especially the smaller diffuse colloid goitres in children and young persons. A suitable iodine solution is Lugol's iodine, 0.5 ml in water daily. An alternative is to give 60 mg of potassium iodide daily.

Thyroid extract. An adult is given 20 mg of thyroid extract daily by mouth for 2 weeks. The dose is increased by 20-mg increments at fortnightly intervals until a daily dose of 100 mg is reached.

The weight, pulse rate, and if possible the basal metabolic rate (BMR) of the patient should be checked at regular intervals. Weight loss, increased pulse rate and raised BMR are indications of hyperthyroidism, and are a signal to reduce the dosage or stop treatment. This treatment should only be undertaken by a doctor.

Surgical treatment. Very large goitres, especially adenomatous ones, may respond neither to iodine nor thyroid therapy. The only other way then of removing the goitre is by surgery. The operation for removal of goitre is called thyroidectomy.

Conditions associated with goitre

Endemic cretinism, a condition in children, occurs most commonly in endemic goitre areas, and is usually due to iodine deficiency in the mother. The infant may appear normal at birth, but is slow to develop, small in size, mentally dull, has coarse, thick skin and a characteristic face with depressed nose and often a protruding enlarged tongue.

Deaf-mutism (inability to hear and speak), dwarfism, certain mental abnormalities and neuromotor disabilities are markedly more frequent among the children of mothers with goitre (see Fig. 34) and especially

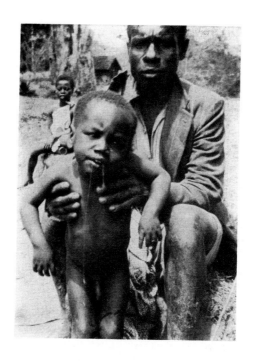

FIGURE 34. Mental deficiency in a child of a goitrous mother.

in areas of high goitre endemicity. It has been shown that, when pregnant women with goitre due to iodine deficiency are given iodine early in pregnancy, their chances of having a cretinous or mentally retarded infant are greatly reduced.

A person with goitre is more liable to develop symptoms and signs due to excessive secretion (hyperthyroidism) and diminished secretion (hypothyroidism) of thyroxine than a non-goitrous person. Similarly, carcinoma (cancer) of the thyroid gland more commonly occurs in those with goitre.

Benign goitres, especially if large, adenomatous, or situated low in the neck, may cause pressure symptoms, such as difficulty in breathing, persistent cough, and voice change.

Prevention

Where goitre is prevalent, it constitutes a public-health problem and should be tackled as such. Goitres may be unsightly and may result in any of the conditions described above. The possibility of even a small percentage of the children of goitrous mothers being cretinous, deaf mutes or mentally retarded is important and worthy of action. Rather than try to treat every sufferer in the community, it is far better to try to prevent the occurrence of goitre. This can most satisfactorily be achieved by the addition of iodine to all salt that is sold in an area. Salt is used as a vehicle for iodization because it is a product almost universally purchased and consumed. Thus if only iodized salt is sold in a district, it can be assumed that all the inhabitants will be getting sufficient iodine. However, in those parts of Africa where rural dwellers dig or make their own salt, the sale of iodized salt will not solve the problem.

Iodization of salt will reduce the size of many existing goitres and will prevent them from occurring in the future. Salt is most commonly iodized by the addition of potassium or sodium iodide, but potassium iodate is preferable in the climate that prevails in much of Africa. The amount added should be enough to provide about 1 part of iodine to 20 000 parts of salt, although this will depend on the amount of salt consumed in any given area.

In areas where goitre is endemic it is preferable that legislation be introduced to ensure that only iodized salt is sold. Iodization of salt has proved extremely effective in preventing goitre in Switzerland, parts of the United States, Colombia and elsewhere.

Where iodization of salt is impracticable, the use of injections of iodized oil as a preventive measure should be considered.

In areas where goitre has been proved to be due to goitrogens in the diet, it can be prevented by omitting from the diet the item of food responsible.

21. NUTRITIONAL ANAEMIAS

Anaemia is an important and very prevalent disease in Africa. There are numerous ways of classifying anaemia, some based on the cause of the disease. These are fully discussed in standard textbooks of medicine.

Anaemias of nutritional origin are due most commonly to a deficiency of iron or protein, or both; they are due less often to folate (folic acid) deficiency. Iron deficiency in the body is frequently due to a failure to absorb iron present in the food rather than to a low total iron content of the diet, and also to an increased loss of iron due to many conditions, the most important of which is severe infestation with hookworms. The importance of iron deficiency as a cause of anaemia in children and in women during pregnancy and lactation has been discussed on p. 69-71. Macrocytic anaemias due to vitamin B_{12} and folic acid deficiencies are mentioned on p. 83-85. Folate deficiency is especially prevalent in pregnant women.

144

Causes

A person has anaemia when his blood has less haemoglobin than normal. Haemoglobin is present in the red blood cells as a red pigment made of protein with iron linked to it. In anaemia either the amount of haemoglobin in each red cell is low (hypochromic anaemia) or there is a reduction in the total number of red cells in the body. The life of each red cell is about 4 months, and so the red bone marrow is constantly manufacturing new cells to allow for replacement. This process requires protein, minerals and vitamins, all of which must originate in food consumed.

Protein. This is needed both for the framework of the red blood cells and for the manufacture of the haemoglobin to go with it.

Minerals. Iron is essential for the manufacture of haemoglobin, and if sufficient is not available, the cells produced will be smaller and each will have less haemoglobin than normal. Copper and cobalt are other mineral elements necessary, in small amounts.

Vitamins. Vitamin B_{12} and folic acid are necessary for the normal manufacture of red blood cells. Ascorbic acid (vitamin C) also plays a role in blood formation.

The normal child at birth has a high haemoglobin level (usually at least 125 percent of the accepted norm for infants, or 18 g/100 ml) but during the first few weeks many cells are haemolysed. The iron liberated is not lost but is stored in the body, especially in the liver and spleen. As milk is a poor source of iron, this reserve store is used during the early months of life to help increase the volume of blood, which is necessary as the baby grows. This store plus the small quantity of iron supplied in breast milk is sufficient for perhaps 6 months, but after that it is desirable that other iron-containing foods enter the diet. At birth a premature infant has a reduced number of red blood cells, and so it will be much more prone to anaemia. Similarly, iron deficiency in the mother may affect these vital stores and render the infant more liable to anaemia.

After 6 months, if the infant continues to live entirely on breast milk (as is not uncommon in some parts of Africa), he will be receiving insufficient iron to allow for a normal increase in the volume of blood, and anaemia will result. This is a common cause of anaemia in children 6 to 12 months of age. It cannot be remedied by dried skim milk or any ordinary milk powder, for these have a low content of iron (unless the product is specially enriched with iron, in which case the label on the package or tin should state that iron has been added). Although it is desirable that breast-feeding should continue well beyond 6 months, it is also necessary that other foods containing iron should be introduced into the diet at this time.

After complete weaning from the breast, the child between 1 and 2 years of age will often be receiving a mainly carbohydrate diet. Under these circumstances he may be getting sufficient iron, but probably insufficient protein to maintain a normal haemoglobin level.

However, although most solid diets, both for children and adults, provide sufficient iron for normal needs, large numbers of the community have increased needs. This may be due to blood loss from hookworm or bilharzia infections, to loss at menstruation or during childbirth, or from wounds. Women have increased needs during pregnancy for the foetus and during lactation to supply the iron present in breast milk. It is stressed that iron from vegetable products, including cereal grains, is less well absorbed than that from most animal products.

For the above reasons it will be clear that anaemia is common in premature infants; in young children over 6 months of age on a purely milk diet; in women rather than in men, especially during pregnancy and lactation; in persons infected with certain parasites; and in those who get only marginal quantities of iron, mainly from vegetable foods.

Diagnosis

Haemoglobin is necessary to carry oxygen, and many of the symptoms and signs of anaemia mentioned below are due to the reduced capacity of the blood to transport oxygen.

These symptoms are:

- Tiredness;
- Pallor of the mucous membranes and beneath the nails;
- Palpitations — the subject complains of being aware of his heartbeat;
- Breathlessness following even normal exertion;
- Oedema (in chronic, severe cases).

A preliminary diagnosis may be made by examining the tongue, the conjunctiva of the lower eyelid, and the nailbed, all of which appear paler than normal.

An inexperienced examiner can compare the redness of these sites in the patient with those of a normal person, for example, his assistant or himself. Enlargement of the heart (cardiomegaly) is not frequently seen even in severe anaemia in Africans.

Diagnosis can be confirmed by measuring the haemoglobin level in the blood by one of many methods available. These range in simplicity (as well as accuracy) from the Tallquist method (a drop of blood from the fingertip or ear lobe is placed on special paper and the colour compared with that of a colour scale) to electrophoresis which can normally be performed only in a large laboratory. A useful test is the measurement of the haematocrit level. This is done by placing blood in a capillary tube and spinning it in a special centrifuge, which separates the red cells from the plasma. If the haematocrit and haemoglobin levels are known then it is possible to calculate the mean cell haemoglobin concentration. A haemoglobin level below 12 g/100 ml in an adult woman and below 13 g in a man is considered abnormally low. Serum ferritin levels, which can be measured only in very sophisticated laboratories, provide a good indication of iron stores in the body.

Treatment

The treatment used for anaemia will depend on the cause. When in doubt, both iron and protein should be prescribed. For anaemia in pregnant women, folate should also be given.

In iron deficiency anaemia, adults should receive 200-250 mg of ferrous sulphate in tablet form three times a day, the dose being determined by the ferrous sulphate content of the tablets. Children should receive a ferrous sulphate mixture in a dose of 50 mg ferrous sulphate per day per year of age. In patients who are vomiting or extremely ill, iron dextran can be given by intramuscular injection for a few days. Adults receive 5 ml (50 mg per ml) daily or on alternate days. Children receive proportionately less.

The anaemia of children with obvious protein deficiency will not respond to iron alone, and dried skim milk (enriched with vitamin A, see p. 103) or some other protein-containing substance must be given. In many cases of anaemia (in adults) in tropical Africa, protein will be of benefit. In macrocytic anaemias in which the blood cells are enlarged, response to folic acid or vitamin B_{12} is usually good. If hookworm ova are present in the stools an appropriate anthelmintic should of course be given. Ascorbic acid (vitamin C) will enhance the absorption of iron from food.

Numerous other anaemias are important in tropical Africa, but they are not strictly nutritional in origin. They are dealt with in most standard textbooks of medicine.

147

22. NUTRITIONAL NEUROPATHIES

The nervous system is the communications system within the body, and is a highly complicated mechanism. If it does not function properly, there can be important consequences. The nervous system needs oxygen and nutrients, and obtains its energy from carbohydrates. A range of complex enzymes controls its functioning. These enzymes are proteins and their activities require the participation of a number of vitamins. It is not surprising therefore that dietary deficiencies can cause symptoms and signs indicating impairment or damage to the nervous system.

The relationship between diet and the nervous system is still not fully understood and the subject is beyond the scope of this book. Nevertheless it is important for all medical persons to keep in mind that any disease of the nervous system may have a nutritional origin. If it is impossible to obtain a proper diagnosis of a nutritional disease, the sufferer should be advised and assisted to get a balanced diet.

The B group of vitamins has a special place in relation to the nervous system. As will be seen in Chapter 24, these vitamins are commonly found in the outer layers of cereal grains. Milling tends to reduce the quantity of B vitamins in cereal flours. Deficiencies of B vitamins are therefore becoming more common in Africa, and cases of various neuropathies are likely to increase. For example, the author encountered an outbreak of a neuropathy in a Tanzanian institution that was caused by a change in diet from lightly milled to highly milled maize-meal as the main source of energy.

Neuropathies may lead to weakness and pins-and-needles in the feet, severe burning pains, ataxia, nerve deafness, disturbances of vision, absent or exaggerated reflexes, etc. There is much overlapping in the causation of many of these conditions, and classification is difficult. Davidson (1972) details the conditions mentioned, and gives the following simple classification:

Group I. Where the lesion is predominantly in the peripheral nerves. This group includes:

- The polyneuropathies of beriberi (see p. 93-95), alcoholism and pregnancy;
- The "burning feet" syndrome.

Group II. Where the lesion is predominantly in the central nervous system. This group includes:

- Wernickes' encephalopathy;

- Nutritional amblyopia;
- The cord syndromes — spinal ataxia; spastic paraplegia and lathyrism; subacute combined degeneration (vitamin B_{12} deficiency).

23. MINOR NUTRITIONAL DISORDERS

The most important and serious diseases resulting from nutritional deficiencies have already been covered. These have been described in terms of syndromes or disease entities, and have not been classified according to their aetiology. There are other clinical conditions that are due to deficiencies of the diet, some of which may later lead to the diseases described earlier. Some are physical signs that can be observed, but that cause little disfigurement or disability. Some are conditions that have a specific known aetiology. Others occur commonly in malnourished persons, yet the exact cause has not been elucidated.

All are of some importance and should be looked for because they can lead a medical worker into an investigation of the diet of a patient, and can thus serve to prevent the onset of more serious disease. They should especially be sought when examining groups of persons routinely, such as in schools, prisons and institutions, or during medical surveys of a community. It is these minor disorders that can serve as indicators of the dietary status of the community as a whole.

Night blindness

In night blindness, ability to see in dim light is reduced to well below average. Apparatus and special tests have been evolved to assess this condition. In African children the mother may notice that the child fails to recognize her when in a dimly lit, windowless hut. Night blindness is not a serious disability, except in persons like drivers and those working with machinery on night shifts in factories. However, it is caused by lack of vitamin A, and is therefore a very important early warning that the individual may develop more serious signs of vitamin A deficiency, in particular xerophthalmia.

Dry scaly skin or xerosis

Normal skin is smooth, slightly oily and has a healthy sheen. In xerosis, the skin loses these characteristics, and becomes dry, scaly and rather rough to the touch. Pieces of the skin tend to flake off in a way similar to dandruff of the scalp. This condition is thought to be due mainly to vitamin A deficiency. However, lack of protein and fat may also play a part.

Crazy-pavement, or cracked skin (mosaic dermatosis)

This is commonly found on the lower leg. The skin resembles a paved walk or the sun-baked and cracked bed of a dried-up mud swamp. There are islands of fairly normal skin, each surrounded by a shallow crack. The edges may be scaly or desquamating. Protein and vitamin A deficiency may play a part in its causation; dirt and alternate exposure to dryness and moisture under hot conditions may also be causative factors.

Follicular hyperkeratosis

Type I follicular hyperkeratosis consists of lesions, most commonly seen on the backs of the arms. The lesions feel spiky to the touch and consist of multiple horny dry papules, which on close inspection are seen to

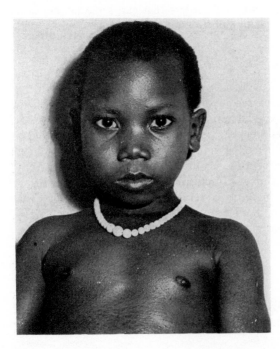

FIGURE 35. Follicular hyperkeratosis. It is seen here as a fine papular eruption.

150

arise from a hair follicle. This condition is associated with a deficiency of vitamin A and possibly also of riboflavin.

Type II follicular hyperkeratosis is similar in appearance and occurs commonly on the trunk or thighs (see Fig. 35). The surrounding skin is less dry and the mouths of the hair follicles are seen to contain brown-pigmented denatured blood. This is possibly due to vitamin C deficiency.

Dyssebacea (naso-labial seborrhoea)

This condition, in which plugs of yellowish keratin stand out from the follicles, is usually seen on each side of the nose, but sometimes extends to other parts of the face (see Fig. 36). It is believed to be due to riboflavin deficiency.

Angular stomatitis

This develops at the angles or corners of the mouth as fissures or cracks radiating from the angle of the mouth onto the skin (see Fig. 37). Some-

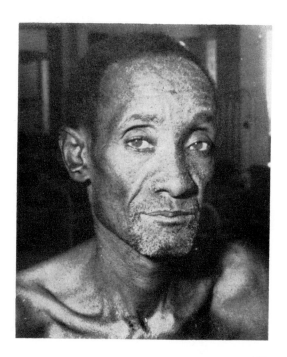

FIGURE 36. Dyssebacea or naso-labial seborrhoea seen especially on the nose and forehead. It consists of tiny raised plugs of keratin standing out from the follicles.

151

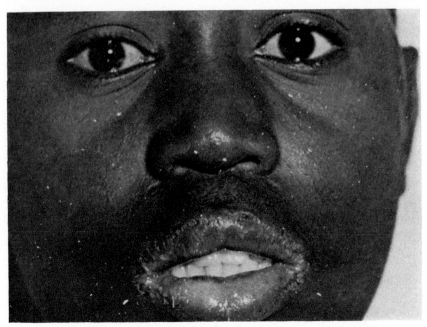

FIGURE 37. Angular stomatosis and cheilosis.

times the cracks extend onto the mucous membrane inside the mouth. These cracks have a raw appearance, but may become yellowish due to secondary infection. Angular stomatitis is especially associated with riboflavin deficiency. Niacin and pyridoxine deficiency may also be involved.

Cheilosis

In cheilosis, cracks, which may be either red and sore or dry and healing, occur on both lips. Sometimes the lips are rather red with a generalized thinning of the epithelium. Deficiency of riboflavin and possibly of other vitamins may be the cause. Cheilosis frequently occurs in conjunction with angular stomatitis, and is easily confused with cracked lips caused by particular weather conditions, especially dry cold winds.

Scrotal (or genital) dermatitis

The skin of the scrotum (or the genital region in females) is affected, becoming dry and irritated. There may be desquamation, intense itching

152

and secondary infection. Riboflavin deficiency (and possibly deficiency of other B vitamins) seems to be the cause.

Bitot's spots

These occur in both eyes and are seen on the outer edge of the cornea. The spots consist of triangular-shaped, raised white plaques (see Fig. 38). When examined closely, they look like a fine foam with many tiny white bubbles. This foamy material is soft and can be wiped away. In Africans, they are often surrounded by a brown-pigmented area. These lesions are associated with vitamin A deficiency in young children.

Conjunctival xerosis

This condition is seen as a drying of the conjunctiva (xerosis) which has lost its shininess and lustre. Instead of being like a clean piece of reflecting glass, the surface is smoky and dull and no longer reflects light. The conjunctiva is often wrinkled and may be thickened. This condition is a sign of vitamin A deficiency and, if not treated, may lead to keratomalacia and blindness (see p. 103).

FIGURE 38. Bitot's spots. *Left:* Note brown pigmented area surrounding spots located on the temporal side of the cornea. *Right:* Under magnification spots appear as small white foam-bubbles.

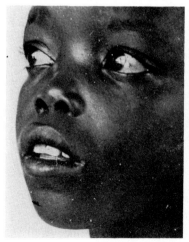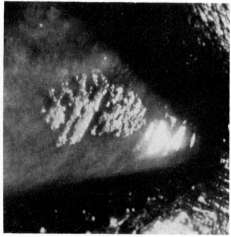

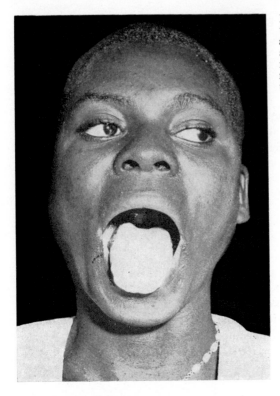

FIGURE 39. Oedema of the tongue. The tongue is swollen and has caused pressure against the teeth. This has resulted in the indentation or notches seen on the sides of the tongue.

Oedema of the tongue

The tongue is swollen, with notches on the sides corresponding to the teeth (see Fig. 39). The papillae are usually prominent. This condition is associated with deficiency of riboflavin and niacin.

Atrophic tongue

The tongue is much smoother than normal, usually reddened (magenta-coloured) and denuded of normal papillae. It may be painful. This condition may be due to lack of niacin.

Patchy glossitis

In patchy glossitis, the tongue shows patchy desquamation in which the patches are often red and inflamed oval areas. This is usually the result

154

of riboflavin deficiency and may sometimes be accompanied by oedema of the tongue.

Parotid swelling

This is seen as a swelling, usually bilateral, just in front of and slightly below the meatus (hole) of the ear. It can be felt as a firm area corresponding to the anatomy of the parotid gland. The swellings may disappear completely after a period on a balanced diet. This condition is possibly associated with protein deficiency.

Tropical ulcers

These ulcers affect the lower leg and may be single or multiple. They are chronic, may be of large size, and are often grossly infected. The cause has not been fully elucidated, but is possibily nutritional. Tropical ulcers are rare in well-nourished persons.

Dental caries (dental decay)

Caries and erosion may occur in any of the teeth, and may possibly be linked with poor nutrition. A lack of calcium and vitamin D in childhood has often been incriminated but has not been proved to cause dental caries. Fluorine is necessary for the formation of a dental enamel with maximum resistance to caries. However, factors such as excess consumption of sugar, especially in a form that sticks to the teeth, and poor dental hygiene may play a part. In general, Africans suffer much less from dental caries than do Europeans or Americans. However, urban Africans who abandon traditional diets in favour of westernized diets tend to develop more caries. In Africa, gum disease (gingivitis) may be more important than dental caries as a reason for loss of teeth in adults. In any nutrition survey it is useful to determine in each person the number of teeth that are decayed, missing, and filled.

Vascularization of the cornea

This condition is preceded by the presence of enlarged blood vessels on the conjunctiva surrounding the cornea. These may eventually spread onto the cornea. This is believed to be associated with riboflavin deficiency.

155

A summary of the signs to be looked for in a nutrition examination and the references to the relevant passages in this book are given below.

Part of body examined	Possible changes or disorders	Page reference
Hair	Colour change	116
	Texture change	116
Eyes	Bitot's spots	153
	Xerosis and xerophthalmia	103, 153
	Keratomalacia	103
	Pallor of the conjuctiva of the lower lid	146
	Vascularization of the cornea	155
Mouth	Angular stomatitis	151
	Cheilosis	152
	Glossitis	154
	Atrophic tongue	154
	Oedema of tongue	154
	Mottled teeth	74
	Carious teeth	155
	Swollen or bleeding gums	111
	Pallor of tongue	146
Skin	Oedema	115
	Follicular hyperkeratosis	150
	Crazy-pavement	150
	Dry scaly	149
	Hyperpigmentation	100
	Ulcers	155
	Haemorrhages	111
	Pallor beneath nails	146
Central	Apathy	116
nervous	Irritability	116
system	Anaesthesia or sensory changes	95-97
	Calf tenderness	95-97

Part of body examined	Possible changes or disorders	Page reference
	Abnormal gait	95-97
	Loss of reflexes	95-97
Skeleton	Deformity (e.g., knock-knees)	107
	Rickety rosary	107
	Bony swelling	107
	Skeletal fluorosis	74
Other	Thyroid enlargement	139
	Height	25
	Weight	25
	Haemoglobin	146
	Skinfold thickness (special calipers are necessary)	29
	Arm circumference	29
	Chest circumference	29
	Head circumference	29

At the examination, the name, sex, and age of the individual should be recorded, and, if female, whether she is pregnant or lactating. It is also important that other observations that many have a bearing on the case should be noted, e.g., parasitic infections, and scarred cornea.

TYPE OF DEFICIENCY AND ASSOCIATED SIGNS

A list of deficiency disorders and the references to the relevant pages in this book are given below.

Deficiency	Associated disorder	Page reference
Vitamin A	Follicular hyperkeratosis, type I	150
	Night blindness	149

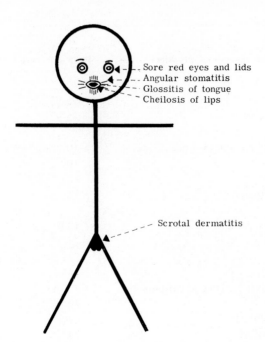

FIGURE 40. Characteristics of riboflavin deficiency (ariboflavinosis).

Sore red eyes and lids
Angular stomatitis
Glossitis of tongue
Cheilosis of lips

Scrotal dermatitis

Deficiency	Associated disorder	Page reference
Vitamin A *(continued)*	Bitot's spots	153
	Conjunctival xerosis	103, 153
	Corneal xerosis	104
	Keratomalacia	103
	Possibly also dry scaly skin and crazy-pavement skin	149
Riboflavin *(sometimes called ariboflavinosis,* Fig. 40)		
	Angular	151
	Cheilosis of lips	152
	Scrotal or genital dermatitis	152
	Possibly also follicular hyperkeratosis,	150
	oedema of the tongue, magenta tongue	154
	and patchy glossitis	154
	Vascularization of the cornea	155

158

Deficiency	Associated disorder	Page reference
Thiamine	Oedema	115
	Anaesthesia	95-97
	Calf tenderness	95-97
	Abnormal gait	95-97
	Various central nervous system signs	148-149
Niacin	Hyperpigmentation	100
	Pellagrous dermatitis	100
	Atrophic tongue	154
Vitamin C	Swollen or bleeding gums	111
	Skin haemorrhages (petechial, etc.)	86, 111
	Other haemorrhages	111
	Follicular hyperkeratosis, type II	150
	Tender subperiosteal swellings	111
Vitamin D	Deformity	107
	Rickety rosary	107
	Bony swelling	107
	Bow legs	107
	Knock-knees	107
Protein (*usually associated with energy deficiency*)	Muscle wasting	115
	Apathy	116
	Irritability	116
	Oedema	115
	Dermatosis	116
	Hair changes	115
	Weight reduction	115
	Height reduction	115
	Small arm-circumference	115
Iodine	Enlargement of thyroid	139
	Cretinism	142
	Deaf-mutism	142
	Mental retardation	142

Deficiency	Associated disorder	Page reference
Fluorine		
● Deficiency	Dental caries	155
● Excess	Mottled teeth	74
	Bone changes	74
Iron	Anaemia	144
	Pale conjunctiva of lower lid	146
	Pallor of tongue	146
	Pallor of nail bed	146

IV. FOODS

24. CEREALS, STARCHY ROOTS
AND OTHER MAINLY CARBOHYDRATE FOODS

Foods with a predominantly carbohydrate content are important because they form the basis of most diets in Africa. They usually provide 70 percent or more of the energy intake of the population; this may be contrasted with the situation in the United States, where often less than 40 percent comes from this source.

Cereals

Many plants from the family of grasses have through the ages been cultivated by man for their edible seeds; these are the cereal grains. In Africa they form an important part of the diet of many people. They include maize, sorghum, millet, wheat, rice, barley, oats and teff.

A new cereal of considerable interest is triticale, a cross between wheat and rye.

Although the shape and size of the seed may be different, all cereal grains have a fairly similar structure and nutritive value; 100 g of whole grain provides about 350 Calories, 8 to 12 g of protein, and useful amounts of calcium, iron (though phytic acid may hinder absorption of these), and the B vitamins. In their dry state they are completely lacking in vitamin C, and, except for yellow maize, they contain no carotene (pro-vitamin A).

To produce a balanced diet, cereals should be supplemented with foods rich in protein, minerals, and vitamins A and C. (Vitamin D can come from exposure of the skin to sunlight.)

Figure 41 illustrates the structure of all cereal grains. The structure consists of:

161

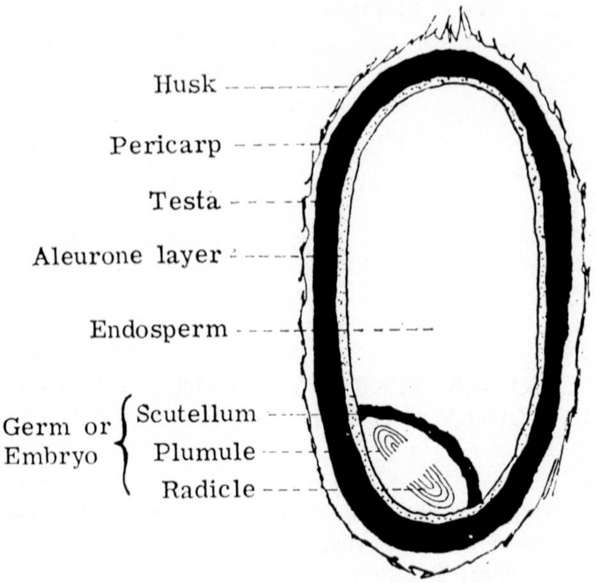

Husk ‒‒‒‒‒‒

Pericarp ‒‒‒‒

Testa ‒ ‒ ‒

Aleurone layer ‒ ‒‒‒

Endosperm ‒ ‒ ‒

Germ or { Scutellum ‒‒‒
Embryo { Plumule ‒‒‒
{ Radicle ‒‒‒

FIGURE 41. Cross-section of a wheat kernel.

● The *husk* of cellulose, which has no nutritive value for humans;

● The *pericarp* and *testa*, two rather fibrous layers containing few nutrients;

● The *aleurone layer*, which is rich in protein, vitamins and minerals;

● The *embryo* or *germ*, consisting of the *plumule* and *radicle* attached to the grain by the *scutellum*. The embryo is very rich in nutrients, and is the part of the grain that sprouts if the grain is planted or soaked in water;

● The *endosperm*, comprising more than half of the grain and consisting mainly of starch.

It should be noted that although small in size the embryo often contains 50 percent of the thiamine, 30 percent of the riboflavin, and 30 percent of the niacin of the whole grain; the aleurone and other outer coats contain 50 percent of the niacin and 35 percent of the riboflavin. Thus the endosperm, although by far the largest part of the grain, often contains only one third or less of the B group of vitamins. It is also poorer than the other parts in protein and minerals.

162

Milling. The above points have been stressed because cereal grains are subjected to many different processes during preparation for human consumption. All of the processes are designed to remove the fibrous layers of the grain. Some, however, also attempt to produce a highly refined white product consisting mainly of endosperm. All these processes reduce the nutritional value of the grain.

Traditional methods involving the use of a pestle and mortar (*kinu*) or stones usually produce a cereal grain that has lost some of its outer coats, but has retained at least part of the germ including the scutellum. Although very careful and prolonged preparation using traditional methods can yield a highly refined product, such preparation is unusual. Light milling, similar to home-pounding, also produces a product that retains most of the nutrients; mechanization of this type takes a great burden off the woman of the household.

Heavy milling to produce a highly refined product is undesirable from a nutritional point of view. Highly milled cereals such as white maize flour (*sembe*), polished rice and white wheat flour have lost most of the germ and outer layers, and with them most of the B vitamins and some of the protein and minerals.

Millers are, however, servants of the public, and the public increasingly demands products that are pure white, have a bland, neutral taste, and are easily digestible. These demands have led in recent years to a vast increase in the production of highly refined cereal flours and white rice. The millers have responded to public demand by devising "improved" milling machinery that separates more and more of the nutritious parts from the grain, leaving the white endosperm.

In urban areas, where wheat is being increasingly used, the bakers have encouraged this trend because white wheat flour has better baking qualities. The trader also prefers the highly milled product because it stores better. Its low fat content reduces the chances of rancidity and its low vitamin content makes it less attractive to insects and other pests.

In many countries food fashions begin with the wealthier people and in Africa these have often been the immigrants. As long as the new food fashion remains confined to those with a high income it need do no harm, for they can afford a better all-round diet. However, the white-flour fashion has spread first to the wage-earners, and, more recently, to the farmer.

This swing away from tradition toward false sophistication could cause much harm. Where it leads to the consumption of a staple cereal rendered deficient by milling, widespread ill-health could result among those who do not include in their diet other foods that make up for this deficiency. It would be a tragedy to see in the last quarter of the twentieth century in Africa a repetition of the misery, suffering and death that

163

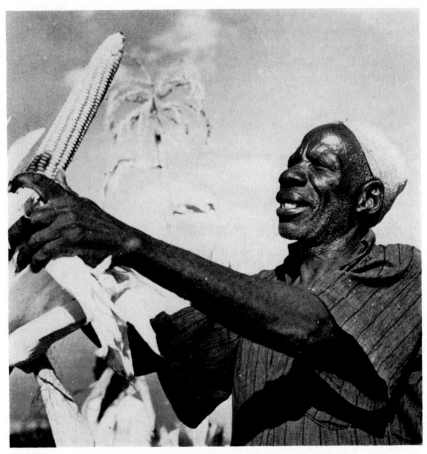

FIGURE 42. A farmer inspects his maize crop.

resulted directly from the introduction of milled cereals to the people of Asia in the nineteenth century.

With the increase of industrialization and urbanization there is a tendency toward a much greater use of bread because of its convenience for workers eating away from home. This trend should be noted and the feasibility of a combination of cereal flours investigated.

Manufactured cereal products are being increasingly sold as baby and breakfast foods. These are mainly imported. They may be convenient but they are relatively expensive and have no inherent advantage, from a nutritional point of view, over local cereals prepared in a traditional manner. Yet they may be highly advertised, be considered as prestige foods, and falsely regarded as more nutritious than local foods. Their

164

use should in general be discouraged for those who cannot really afford them.

Maize or corn. The cultivation of maize began in America. Seeds were brought to Europe and later to Africa, where maize now forms the most important part of the diet of many areas (see Fig. 42). The popularity of maize is due to the fact that it gives a high yield per unit area, it grows in warm and fairly dry areas (much drier than those needed for rice, though not as dry as for sorghum and millet), it matures rapidly and has a natural resistance to bird damage. The maize grains contain quantities of protein (10 percent) similar to other cereals, but much of this is in the form of zein, a poor-quality protein containing only small amounts of lysine and tryptophan. The association noted between maize consumption and pellagra (see Chapter 15) may be due to a deficiency of these amino acids. Whole-grain maize contains 2 mg niacin/100 g, less than wheat or rice, and about the same as oats (see p. 82). New varieties of maize have now been developed with an improved amino-acid pattern, for example *opaque-2* maize, but this is not yet widely grown in Africa. However, a type of maize that is naturally rich in lysine and tryptophan does occur in Africa.

Milling reduces the nutritive value of maize just as it does with other cereals. The increased popularity and use of highly milled maize-meal (*sembe*) as opposed to traditionally ground or lightly milled maize (*dona*) are creating a problem, since *sembe* is deficient in B vitamins. The vitamin B content of maize, in mg/100 g, is shown below.

Item	Thiamine	Riboflavin	Niacin
Maize, whole-grain	0.35	0.13	2.0
Maize, lightly milled (*dona*)	0.3	0.13	1.5
Maize, 65 percent extraction, highly milled (*sembe*)	0.05	0.03	0.6

These data show that it is necessary to eat 600 g *sembe* to obtain the same amount of thiamine as is present in 100 g of *dona*, yet *sembe* is the more expensive.

The vitamin B constituents lost in milling may be replaced in maize meal or other cereal flours by adding vitamin preparations up to certain desired levels. Enrichment of this kind has been effective in many countries. Legislation to ensure an adequate level of B vitamins in cereal flours may be a feasible and worthwhile procedure for African countries to adopt.

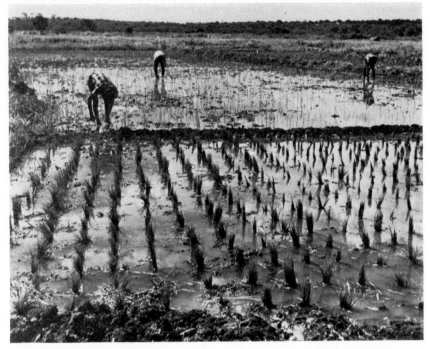

FIGURE 43. Rice-growing in East Africa.

Rice. Rice, like other cereals, is a domesticated grass, wild varieties of which have existed for centuries in both Asia and Africa. (The Asiatic cultivation method of transplanting into flooded basins is used in Africa; see Fig. 43.) The outer layers and the germ of the rice grain together contain nearly 80 percent of the thiamine, whereas the endosperm, though constituting 90 percent of the weight, contains less than 10 percent of the thiamine. Lysine and threonine are the limiting amino acids in rice.

The traditional African method of pounding rice in a wooden mortar and winnowing it in a shallow tray usually results in the loss of about half of the outer layers and germ, and leaves a product containing about 0.25 mg thiamine/100 g (slightly less than *dona*).

The milling and subsequent polishing of rice to produce the highly esteemed white rice on sale in the shops remove nearly all the outer layers and germ, and leave a product containing only about 0.06 mg thiamine/100 g (similar to *sembe*). This is grossly deficient. In Asia, many poor persons eat nothing but rice for much of the year. A person eating 500 g of highly milled polished rice (just over 1 lb) per day would only get 0.3 mg thiamine. The same quantity of home-pounded or lightly

166

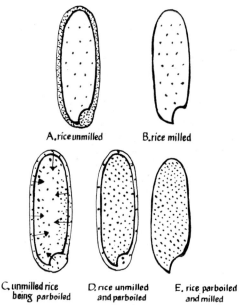

A. rice unmilled   B. rice milled

C. unmilled rice   D. rice unmilled   E. rice parboiled
being parboiled   and parboiled   and milled

FIGURE 44. The milling and parboiling of rice. Each black dot denotes a particle of thiamine. In unmilled rice (A) this is mainly in the outer layers and germ. When milled (B), the rice grain is left with little thiamine. During the process of parboiling (C) the thiamine is drawn into the endosperm (D) and if the rice is now milled and the outer layer removed a grain is left containing adequate quantities of thiamine (E).

milled rice would provide approximately 1.25 mg thiamine, which is about the normal requirement for an average man.

When discussing maize it was mentioned that legislation to require millers to put additional vitamins into cereal flours could be effective. This system does not work as well with rice because it is bought and eaten in its granular form, whereas maize and wheat and most other cereals are bought as a flour. Attempts have been made in the Far East to add vitamins in a concentrated form to a few artificial granules and then to mix these with the rest of the rice. This has not proved entirely successful, partly because one of the B vitamins, riboflavin, is yellow and this is not acceptable to those who want a uniformly white product.

However, there is a way of providing a highly milled rice that is reasonably white and yet contains adequate quantities of B vitamins. This is by the process of parboiling, usually done in the mill though it can be done in the home: the paddy, or unhusked rice (*mpunga*) is usually steamed. Water is absorbed by the whole grain, including the endosperm, and the B vitamins, which are water soluble, become evenly distributed throughout the whole grain (see Fig. 44). The paddy is dried and dehusked, and is then ready for milling in the ordinary way. Even if highly milled and polished, it still retains the major part of its thiamine and other B vitamins.

At present in Africa, those who eat rice as their staple food either grow and home-pound it themselves, or can afford to buy both highly milled rice and other constituents of a more varied diet. Nevertheless, with the increasing popularity of rice, beriberi could become more common in Africa. The simplest and most effective way of preventing this would be to parboil all rice at the mill.

The fact that the B vitamins are soluble has its disadvantages. Rice that is washed in water too thoroughly loses some of the B vitamins, which are dissolved out. Similarly if rice is boiled in excess water, a considerable proportion of the B vitamins is likely to be discarded in the water after the rice has been cooked. Rice should therefore always be cooked in just the amount of water it will absorb. Any water left over should be used for a soup or stew, since it will contain valuable B vitamins, which should not be wasted.

Wheat. Wheat is grown in the highland areas of East Africa, where for some it is an important food. In many other parts of Africa, where it is not possible to grow wheat, it is imported and is becoming an increasingly important part of the diet, especially of the urban population and the salaried classes. Importation of wheat naturally causes a drain on a country's foreign exchange.

Wheat is usually ground and made into a flour; as with other milled cereals, the nutrient content depends on the degree of milling, i.e., the extraction rate. The extraction rate is the percentage of the original grain that remains in the flour after milling. Thus an 85 percent extraction flour contains 85 percent by weight of the whole grain, 15 percent having been removed. Therefore a high-extraction flour has lost little of the nutrients in the outer coats and germ, whereas a low-extraction flour has lost much.

The advantages of low-extraction flours over high-extraction flours, from the trade point of view, are that they: are whiter, and so more popular; have less fat, and hence less tendency to become rancid; have less phytic acid, which possibly means that minerals from associated foods are absorbed better; have better baking qualities.

The disadvantages of low-extraction flours to the consumer are that they have a lower content of B vitamins, minerals, protein, and roughage or fibre than high-extraction flours.

From the nutritional and economic standpoints, consideration should be given to mixing wheat flour with indigenous cereals or even with cassava flour. The limiting amino acid in wheat is lysine.

FIGURE 45. Weaver
bird on sorghum.

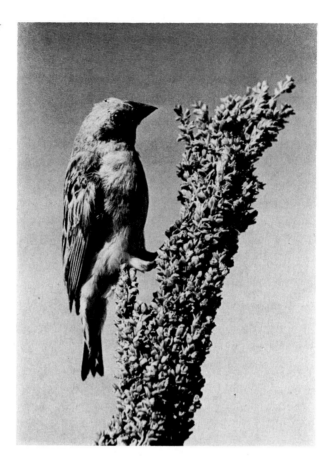

Millets and sorghums. Millets and sorghums are cereal grains widely
grown in Africa and elsewhere. They survive drought conditions better
than maize and other cereals, and so are commonly grown in areas where
rainfall is low or unpredictable.

They are valuable food crops because they nearly all contain a higher
percentage than maize of better protein with a fairly high content of
tryptophan. They are also rich in calcium and iron. Because they tend
to be ground at home and not in the mill, they are less frequently subjected to vitamin, mineral and protein loss. However, in many areas,
they are being partially replaced by irrigated rice and maize, although
they usually continue to be grown for making beer.

Many millets and sorghums have the disadvantage of being attacked
by small birds (see Fig. 45) and also of having a tendency to shed their
grain.

169

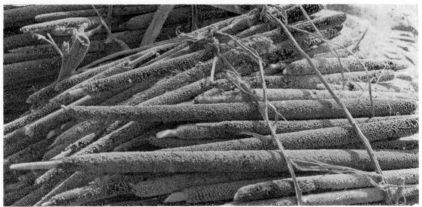

FIGURE 46. Bundles of bulrush millet.

There are several species of millet and sorghum. The three most important in Africa are:

Bulrush millet (*uwele, Pennisetum typhoideum*). As the name implies, this millet looks rather like a bulrush, but the inflorescence may be much longer and thicker, sometimes 1 m × 8 cm (see Fig. 46).

Finger millet (*ulesi, Eleusine coracana*). The inflorescence of this type is shaped like a rather flaccid hand. The seeds are smaller than those of bulrush millet. It is very commonly used for making beer.

Sorghum, guinea corn or *durra* (*mtama, Sorghum vulgare*). There are many varieties of sorghum, most of which grow tall and have a large inflorescence; there are also dwarf varieties. The grain is usually large but varies in colour and shape with the type. Sorghum requires more moisture than millet, but less than maize. Sorghum is a nutritious food since many varieties have a higher protein content than other cereals.

Oats. Oats are not important in African diets. The crop is grown in a few cold highland areas, where it is locally prepared and not usually milled. Oats are a good cereal containing rather more protein than maize, rice, or wheat, but they also contain a considerable quantity of phytic acid, which may hinder absorption of calcium. Oatmeal is imported for porridge making and is used in some manufactured infant foods.

Rye. Rye is little grown in Africa, and even in Europe is not an important item of the diet.

Barley. Barley is grown in some of the wheat-growing districts of Africa. In these places it is usually consumed, after home preparation, as a stiff

170

porridge or *ugali*. In Europe it is now used mainly for animal feeding and in the preparation of alcoholic beverages such as beer and whisky.

Triticale. This new "man-made" cereal is a cross between wheat and rye. It has great promise of high yields and good nutritive value. It is particularly suited to temperate climates.

Teff. Teff (*Eragrostis tef*) is an important cereal in Ethiopia, where it is held in special regard, although it gives a relatively low yield per unit area. It is usually ground into a flour, cooked and eaten as *injera*, a type of baked pancake. The nutritive value of teff is similar to that of other cereal grains, except that it is richer in iron and calcium. The high consumption of teff in parts of Ethiopia may be an important reason why iron-deficiency anaemia is rare there.

Starches and starchy roots

A number of edible tubers, roots and corms form an important part of the diet of many peoples in different parts of the world. In Africa cassava, sweet potatoes, taro (cocoyams), yams and arrowroot are the most important foods in this class. In the cooler parts of the continent the common potato is also widely grown.

These food crops are usually easy to cultivate and give high yields per hectare; they contain large quantities of starch and are therefore a fairly easily obtainable source of food energy. As a staple foodstuffs, however, they are inferior to cereals, because they consist of about two-thirds water and contain much less protein, usually less than 2 percent as against about 10 percent in cereals, although taro and yam contain up to 6 percent of good-quality protein. They also have lower contents of minerals and vitamins.

Cassava. Although cassava (*Manihot esculenta*, or manioc) originated in South America, it is now widely grown in many parts of Africa. Readily established from cuttings, it will grow in poor soil, requires relatively little attention, withstands adverse weather conditions, and is not greatly afflicted by pests or disease. In spite of these favourable qualities, cassava has the great disadvantage of containing little but carbohydrate. It fills the stomach and produces energy but, unless other foods are eaten, the consumer is likely to suffer from deficiency conditions. It is especially unsuitable as the main source of energy for the infant or young child because of its low protein content. It should therefore be supplemented liberally with cereals and also with legumes or other protein-rich foods.

171

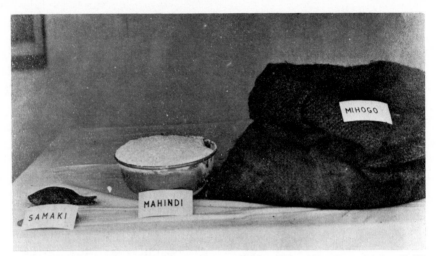

FIGURE 47. One small dried fish *(samaki)* weighing 150 g (5 oz) or 1.4 kg (3 lb) of maize *(mahindi)* contains the same quantity of protein as 6.8 kg (15 lb) of cassava *(mihogo)*.

Cassava contains less than 1 percent of protein as opposed to 10 percent of protein in maize and other cereals (see Fig. 47). It is therefore not surprising that kwashiorkor due to protein deficiency is much more common in young children weaned onto cassava rather than millet or maize. Cassava also has considerably less iron and B vitamins than the cereal grains.

Cassava sometimes contains a cyanogenic glucoside. This poisonous substance is present mainly near the outer coat of the tuber; careful peeling and special soaking methods have been developed by different peoples to remove it.

Cassava leaves are frequently used as a green vegetable. These have a nutritive value similar to other dark green leaves and are an extremely valuable source of carotene (vitamin A), vitamin C, iron and calcium. They also contain some protein. In order to preserve the maximum quantity of vitamin C, the leaves should not be cooked for longer than about 20 minutes.

The tubers may be eaten roasted or boiled, but more often they are sun-dried after soaking, and then made into a powdery white flour. This is usually cheaper than maize or wheat flour, and is not infrequently used to adulterate these products. It is also used by some overseas firms in biscuit making. In West Africa it is used to make *fufu* (a boiled, mashed product).

In non-arid areas, where the main food and nutrition problems are due to a total shortage of food and a deficient energy intake, cassava should be encouraged, because of its high yields and other agricultural advantages.

Sweet potatoes. Sweet potatoes originated in America and are widely grown in tropical Africa, usually from stem cuttings. Like cassava, the irregularly shaped, variously sized tubers contain little protein. They contain some vitamin C, and the coloured varieties, especially the yellow ones, provide useful quantities of carotene (vitamin A). Sweet-potato leaves are often eaten and have very similar properties to cassava leaves. However, as with other tuber crops, the leaves should not be picked to excess since this may reduce the yield of tubers.

Yams. There are innumerable varieties of yams, many of which are indigenous to Africa. There are variations in shape, colour and size as well as of cooking quality, leaf structure and palatability. Besides the many domesticated varieties a number of wild varieties are eaten.

Yams are more extensively grown in West than in East Africa. In Nigeria, for example, despite an increase in popularity of cassava, yams are still the most important root crop.

Yams require a warm humid climate and soil rich in organic matter, which limits their cultivation in East Africa.

The proper cultivation of yams requires initial deep digging and subsequent staking of the twining vine-like plant. The work involved is more arduous than for cassava and the yields, though high, are usually a little lower. However, yams usually contain about twice as much protein (2 percent) as cassava, although this is very much less than cereals.

Taro or cocoyams. Taro (*Colocasia* sp.) originated in Asia, but is quite extensively grown in areas where there is a fairly high rainfall spread over much of the year. It is common in forest areas (e.g., in Ashanti country) and on mountain slopes where there is a high precipitation (e.g., Kilimanjaro). It is often grown in association with bananas or plantains (e.g., by the Buganda) and oil palms. The plant has large "elephant ear" leaves. Both the tubers and the leaves are eaten. The nutritive value is similar to cassava. In parts of Africa taro is being replaced by tania (*Xanthosoma* sp.), a somewhat similar but more robust plant that originated in South America. It outyields taro.

Potatoes. Potatoes were first brought to Europe from South America and became a cheap, useful, high-yielding alternative to whatever the main staple in a given area happened to be, just as cassava is replacing cereals in much of Africa today. However, the mistake of relying almost entirely on one crop was emphasized by the great Irish potato famine of the last century. When the potato crop failed over one million people died and even larger numbers emigrated.

From Europe, potatoes came to Africa, where they are grown in high, cool areas. If well cultivated in the right soil and climate, they can give a very high yield per hectare. Like other starchy tubers, they contain only about 2 percent protein, but the protein is of reasonably good quality. Potatoes also provide small quantities of B vitamins and minerals. They contain about 15 mg vitamin C per 100 g, but this amount is reduced in storage. The keeping quality of potatoes is not good, unless they are stored carefully. In Africa the grower often sells most of his crop and eats the remainder over the next few months, storing his cereal crop for the dry season.

Arrowroot. African arrowroot (*Tacca involucrata*) is occasionally grown in areas with adequate rainfall. The roots are eaten in a variety of ways, often roasted or boiled. Their nutritive value is similar to that of potatoes.

Other predominantly carbohydrate foods

Bananas and plantains. Bananas and plantains should, strictly speaking, be discussed with fruits, but from the nutritional point of view they are more appropriately dealt with under starchy foods. It is difficult to differentiate between the many varieties of plantain and of banana. For the purposes of this book plantains may be described as bananas that are picked green and are cooked before eating. Plantains contain more starch and less sugar than bananas, which are eaten raw like other fruits. Bananas and plantains originally grew wild in damp, warm areas of forest. They have probably been used as food by man since earliest times. Bananas and plantains are now cultivated extensively in many of the humid areas of Africa. Some tribes such as the Buganda in Uganda and the Wachagga of Tanzania depend on plantains as their main food. The plantains are picked while green and the skin is peeled off. They are then either roasted and eaten, or, more commonly, cut up and boiled, and eaten with meat, beans or other foods. Plantains are frequently sun-dried and made into a flour. Each 100 g of green bananas or plantains contain 32 g carbohydrate (mainly as starch), 1.2 g protein, 0.3 g fat, and yield 135 Calories. They also have a high water content. The very low protein content explains why kwashiorkor commonly occurs in young children weaned onto a mainly banana diet. Bananas usually contain about 20 mg vitamin C and 120 μg of vitamin A (as β carotene equivalent)/ 100 g. For this reason fresh fruits and vegetables are much less important in the diet of those whose staple food is banana than in the diet of those

174

whose staple is a cereal or root. Bananas are, however, low in their content of calcium, iron, and B vitamins. As bananas supply only 80 Calories/100 g, it will be seen that to provide even, say, 1 500 Calories, about 2 kg (nearly 5 lb) must be eaten.

Sugar. Sugar as sold in the shop is almost 100 percent sucrose and is essentially pure carbohydrate. In Africa nearly all locally produced sugar comes from sugar cane, while in Europe it comes mainly from sugar beet. In areas where much sugar cane is grown, the consumption of sugar or sugar-cane juice (chewed cane) is usually high. In other parts of the world the consumption of sugar tends to rise with economic advancement (in the United Kingdom it is now about 50 kg per head per year, five times greater than 100 years ago). The average consumption per head per year in Tanzania is now about 6 kg, but this also shows signs of increasing. A rise in consumption of sugar has usually been accompanied by a rise in the incidence of certain nutritional diseases and of dental caries. Taken in moderation, sugar is a pleasant luxury, but it should not be consumed at such a high level that it crowds out of the diet other foods that provide proteins, vitamins and minerals. Its consumption might with advantage be checked at about 12 kg per head per year. White sugar contains no vitamins, protein, fat or minerals. It is a good source of energy and many people find that its sweet taste adds to the enjoyment of eating. The yields of energy per hectare of land are very high on productive sugar estates.

Honey. Honey is extensively gathered from wild hives in Africa; more and more hives are being kept, often in hollowed and suspended pieces of tree trunk, in rural areas. The incentive tends to be the high price of beeswax rather than the honey. However, in Africa as in Europe and elsewhere, honey has gained the false reputation of being of especial nutritive value. In fact it contains only sugar (carbohydrate), water and minute traces of other nutrients. Although merely a source of energy, it has aesthetic value as a pleasant food for humans.

25. LEGUMES, NUTS AND OILSEEDS

Legumes or pulses

Beans, peas, lentils and their like belong to the botanical family of *Leguminosae*. Their edible seeds are called legumes or pulses. Agriculturally this group of plants has the advantage of being able to obtain nitrogen from the air and also to add some to the soil, whereas most other plants take nitrogen from the soil and do not replace it. Legumes usually grow best when they can get water early in their growth, and then have a warm dry spell for ripening. They are therefore often planted at the end of the rains, to ripen early in the dry season.

In Africa the seeds are usually left on the plant to reach full maturity, and are then harvested and dried. Some may be picked earlier and eaten while partly green as in Europe and America.

The dried seeds can be kept and stored in much the same way as cereals. Some varieties are liable to attack by weevils and a small amount of money spent on insecticides to prevent this is definitely a sound economic proposition. However, care must be taken that an excess of insecticide is not applied, that it is relatively safe and that the beans are well washed before cooking.

The legumes are very important from a nutritional point of view, because they are a widely available vegetable food that contains good quantities of protein and B vitamins. They usually supplement very well the predominantly carbohydrate diet of the cereal, root, or plantain eater of Africa. The quality of this protein is not as good as that in most animal products because it is deficient in certain essential amino acids. However, when pulses and cereals are both eaten at one meal together, they supply protein containing good quantities of all the amino acids; this protein is of a high quality rather similar to casein, the protein of milk. Legumes also contain some carotene (provitamin A) and ascorbic acid if eaten green. Similarly, dried legumes allowed to sprout before eating have good quantities of ascorbic acid.

It is important in any area to encourage increased production and consumption of whatever legume is already grown and popular. The local people will have a taste for it, and agricultural conditions are usually suitable. This seems more sensible than trying to introduce a new crop such as soybeans, unless there is a very good reason for this.

It is also highly important to try to get beans (and other pulses) introduced into the diet of children at an early age. Children are able to digest beans just as easily as adults are.

Beans, cowpeas, pigeon peas. A wide variety of beans, peas, lentils, grams, etc. are grown in different areas of Africa. Two of the most widely grown varieties indigenous to Africa are cowpeas and pigeon peas. Despite the introduction of many legumes from elsewhere, these two pulses are still of very great importance in African diets. They contain good quantities of a protein that will supplement the protein present in cereal grains.

Cowpeas are herbaceous annual plants that thrive only in warm climates. They are often grown mixed with other crops. There are a number of varieties.

The pigeon pea is a relatively drought-resistant, deep-rooted perennial plant.

The winged bean (*Psophocarpus tetragonolobus*) is another important legume grown in Africa. However, its high nutritional value is not adequately appreciated. It contains about 35 percent protein, much more than ordinary peas and beans, and almost as much as soybeans.

The large number of other legume seeds of various shapes, colours and sizes on sale at the shop or in the market-place in almost any village in Africa is evidence of an appreciation of variety and culinary finesse in the diets. The nutritive value of most of these legumes seeds is fairly similar. They usually contain about 22 percent protein (as opposed to 1 percent in cassava roots and 10 percent in maize), and good quantities of thiamine, riboflavin and niacin; in addition they are richer in iron and calcium than most of the cereals.

Soybeans. Soybeans originated in Asia. Although of a high nutritive value, they play little part in African diets. Much of the small production is exported. Soybeans contain up to 40 percent protein, 18 percent fat and 20 percent carbohydrate; the protein is of a higher biological quality than that from other plant sources. It has not become a popular food, firstly because oilseed rather than edible varieties have been introduced in the past, and secondly because there is little local knowledge of the best methods of preparing the beans for food. People lacking experience with soybeans find them difficult to prepare and cook, but varieties are available that are edible after simple cooking (or even raw). Many methods have been evolved and used in the Far East. It is questionable whether it is worth attempting at this juncture to popularize this good food in Africa. It might instead be wiser to encourage the wider use of the already established legumes that are accepted parts of the diets of most tribes. Where soybeans are grown they should be locally processed into some commodity suitable for use in the country, either as an enrichment to cereal flours, as an infant food, or for institutional and school-feeding purposes. Thus it is being successfully promoted in Zaire both for school feeding (as a biscuit) and as porridge for weanlings. The oil could be exported and the protein-rich residue cake could be utilized in the country; large quantities of a protein-rich food should clearly not be exported from a protein-deficient continent.

Groundnuts (peanuts, monkeynuts). The term "nut" is a misnomer since, although botanically a nut, the groundnut (*karanga*, *Arachis hypogaea*) is a true pulse, a member of the Leguminosae family. It originated in

177

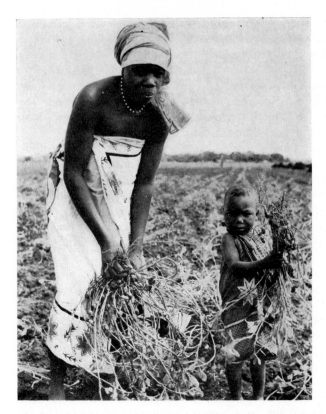

FIGURE 48. This woman and her child are harvesting groundnuts, a food rich in fat, protein and B vitamins. If each person ate a handful of groundnuts per day in addition to their normal diet Africa would be rid of most existing malnutrition.

Brazil, but is now extensively grown in Africa (see Fig. 48). It is an unusual plant in that the flower stalk bearing the ovary burrows into the ground, where a nut containing the seed or seeds develops.

Groundnuts contain much more fat than other legumes, often 45 percent, and also much more niacin (18 mg/100 g) and thiamine, but relatively little carbohydrate (12 percent). The protein content is a little higher than that of most other pulses (27 percent).

Groundnuts are fairly widely grown in Africa. Farmers should produce more for home consumption rather than as cash crops, since they form a very useful addition to the primarily carbohydrate diets of much of tropical Africa. They supply much-needed fat, which is high in energy and assists in the absorption of carotene as well as serving other functions. In predominantly maize diets, groundnuts, with their high content of niacin and also of protein (including the amino acid tryptophan), can in relatively small quantities prevent pellagra. Added to children's diets, their high protein and energy content serves to prevent protein-energy malnutrition. In fact, the simple procedure of adding a handful of ground-

178

nuts per day to the diet of everyone over 6 months of age in Africa would solve a large proportion of the nutritional deficiency problems.

However, groundnuts are all too often grown mainly as a cash crop and sold even in those parts of Africa suffering these problems. They are then usually utilized for oil extraction, and the residue, groundnut cake, is used for animal feed, though it is being increasingly adapted for use as protein-rich human food.

Groundnuts, if damaged during harvesting or if poorly stored in damp conditions, may be attacked by the mould *Aspergillus flavus*. This fungus produces a poisonous toxin known as aflatoxin, which has been shown to cause liver damage in animals and to kill poultry fed on infected groundnuts. It may be toxic also for man, and may be a cause of liver cancer.

Bambara groundnut. The Bambara groundnut (*Voandzeia subterranea*) originated in Africa and is grown widely. It resembles the groundnut in that the flower stalk eventually burrows into the ground where the seed is formed in a round pod. It can survive in moderately sandy soil. However, the Bambara groundnut is not nutritionally similar to the groundnut, having only 6 percent fat but 60 percent carbohydrate. Its protein content of 18 percent is a little lower than most other pulses, but its mineral and vitamin content is similar to that of the bean. This lower fat content means that the crop is not in great demand for oil production. Therefore, instead of being sold as a cash crop, more is used locally for food. With its high content of protein and other nutrients it is a valuable food for children and adults. The Bambara groundnut is one of the most promising pulses in Africa.

Tree nuts

Coconut. Coconut is the most important nut crop in Africa. Its origins are uncertain. The nut, being light and impervious to water, no doubt drifted across many seas to germinate on a new shore. It is now extensively cultivated. The palm tree that bears it is a picturesque and highly useful plant, apart from the food it provides for man (see Fig. 49). The nut when green contains about half a litre of water. This is a very refreshing and hygienic drink, but apart from a little calcium and carbohydrate it has no nutritive value. The white flesh, however, is rich in fat. It is usually sun-dried into copra. The oil from the copra is used both for cooking and for making soap. Copra itself is used in the tropics and elsewhere as an addition to many dishes. Coconut oil has the disadvantage of containing a relatively high proportion of saturated fatty acids.

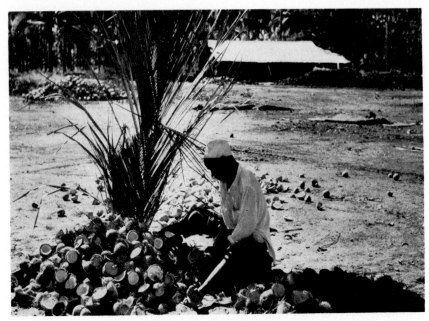

FIGURE 49. The coconut. Its trees provide shade, its husks fuel, its juice refreshment, its copra-oil food or money, and its leaves roofing for houses.

Cashew nut. The cashew nut is produced on a small tree that originated in dry areas of the Americas. It is grown in the drier parts of Africa, and the nuts are mainly exported. They are rich in fat (45 percent) and contain 20 percent protein and 26 percent carbohydrate. The edible swollen stalk of the nut contains good quantities of vitamin C. It is a useful local food but too expensive for most people.

Oilseeds

Sesame. Sesame, or simsim (benniseed in West Africa), is grown fairly widely in both East and West Africa, where it is largely used for oil extraction. The seeds are of various colours and contain about 50 percent fat and 20 percent protein. They are also rich in calcium and contain useful quantities of carotene, iron and B vitamins. They can form a nutritious addition to the diet.

Sunflower seeds. Sunflowers are grown mainly as a cash crop but some of the seeds and some of the oil are eaten locally. The oil has the advantage of being relatively high in polyunsaturated fatty acids. The seeds

180

contain about 36 percent oil (less than sesame), 23 percent protein and some calcium, iron, carotene and B vitamins.

Red palm oil. The product from oil palm (*Elaeis guineensis*) is discussed on page 194.

Other oilseeds. A number of other oil-rich seeds are eaten or used for oil extraction. Those commonly grown in Africa include pumpkin seeds, melon seeds, oyster nut (fluted pumpkin, *Telfairia pedata*) and cottonseed. The last is a major source of oil in the cotton-growing districts of the Sudan, Uganda, Egypt and Tanzania. In West Africa, in addition to some of these East African seeds, shea butter (*Butyrospermum parkii*), butternut (black mango), doumori butter and several other oilseeds are used in the diet. Most of these grow on trees that are indigenous to the region.

26. VEGETABLES AND FRUITS

Vegetables

The term vegetable includes some fruits (e.g., tomatoes and pumpkins), leaves (e.g., amaranth and cabbage), roots (e.g., carrots and turnips), and even stalks (e,g., celery), and flowers (e.g., cauliflower). These differing edible portions come from plants that are often unrelated botanically. However, "vegetable" is a useful term both in nutrition and in domestic terminology.

Vegetables are nearly all eaten soon after they are harvested and are not usually stored for long periods like cereals, tubers, starchy roots, pulses and nuts (there are a few exceptions such as pumpkins and other gourds). In rural Africa, the householder may forage for much of his supply; he usually grows some on his *shamba* or in his backyard, and if he has cash he can buy vegetables in every market and even along the roadside. The African with a low income moving to an urban environment may resent having to purchase vegetables, because he is used to being able to gather wild ones or grow his own. He may therefore spend relatively little on this item of the diet. In any case vegetables are not usually a prestige food, and in few societies are they high on the list of food preferences.

Vegetables are nearly all rich in carotene and vitamin C, and contain significant amounts of calcium, iron, and other minerals. Their content of B vitamins is frequently small. They usually provide only a little energy

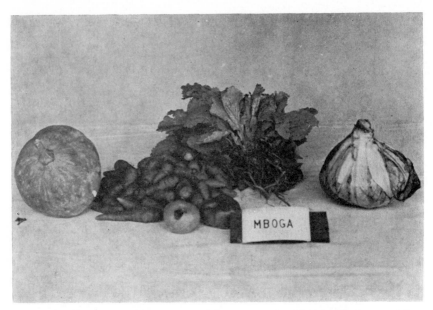

FIGURE 50. Vegetables *(mboga)* are rich in carotene, vitamin C, iron, calcium, and other minerals.

and very little protein. A large proportion of their content consists of indigestible residue, which adds bulk or fibre to the faeces.

In African diets, the dark green leaves are the most valuable vegetables because they contain far more carotene and vitamin C, as well as more protein, calcium and iron than pale green leaves and other vegetables. Thus, amaranth *(mchicha)* is much superior to cabbage or lettuce. Leaves from pumpkin, sweet potato and cassava plants, as well as many wild edible leaves are also excellent.

An increase in the consumption of green leaves and other vegetables could play a major role in ridding Africa of anaemia, which is especially prevalent in women, and in preventing xerophthalmia in children. It would also supply additional calcium and vitamin C, which would prevent the rare disease, scurvy, and might also assist ulcer and wound healing. Vitamin C also enhances iron absorption.

It is not possible here to describe the individual properties of the many vegetables commonly eaten in Africa (see Fig. 50). A few, like pumpkins, can be stored for several months with little loss of nutritive value; others such as leaves and even tomatoes are frequently sun-dried, but a considerable loss of vitamin content occurs. It must also be remembered that the vitamin C content of vegetables is lowered by prolonged cooking.

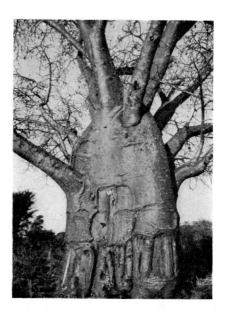

FIGURE 51. Among the variety of wild fruits eaten, that of the baobab *(mbuyu)* is particularly rich in ascorbic acid (vitamin C).

There is no doubt that with growing urbanization and the reduced time for scavenging (because of children attending school and other activities in the village) it is becoming increasingly important that every householder, every village, and every school should devote more time to the growing of vegetables. Often a community garden near the village source of water is a useful adjunct to the villagers' own backyard gardens. In towns, even the smallest piece of land behind a house could, with the assistance of waste water, yield a valuable supply of vegetables all the year round. The allocation of allotment plots for vegetable growing could help solve this problem, and is worthy of serious consideration by town councils and other urban authorities.

Fruits

A wide variety of fruits grow wild (see Fig. 51) or are cultivated in tropical Africa. The varieties available at any one time in a given area depend on the climate, the local tastes for fruit, the species cultivated and the season. The main nutritive value of fruits is their content of vitamin C, which is often high. Some also contain useful quantities of carotene.

Fruits (except the avocado and a few others) contain very little fat or protein, and usually no starch. The carbohydrate is present as various sugars. Fruits, like vegetables, contain much unabsorbable residue mainly as cellulose.

The citrus fruits, such as oranges, lemons, grapefruits, tangerines and limes, contain good quantities of vitamin C, but little carotene. In contrast, papayas, mangoes, and cape gooseberries (*Physalis peruviana*) contain both carotene and vitamin C.

Papayas are useful fruit, especially for those who cultivate a piece of land for a few years and then move on to new land. The papaya grows rapidly and may yield fruit after one or two years. On the other hand, the mango grows slowly, but once established (and it may establish itself) needs no care and yields fruit for half a century. Guavas, which are quite widely grown, contain five times as much vitamin C as do most citrus fruits, and useful amounts of carotene.

The avocado requires special mention because, unlike other fruit, it is rich in fat, a substance that is lacking in many African diets. It could with benefit be much more widely grown and eaten, and fed to children.

The banana, as mentioned earlier, is commonly eaten green in East Africa and is then mainly a starchy food forming the staple diet of many people. When ripe the starch is converted into other sugars. Bananas contain fair quantities of carotene and vitamin C. They are rich in potassium.

A few fruit trees would be a useful addition to all households, both urban and rural.

27. MEAT, FISH, EGGS, MILK AND THEIR PRODUCTS

Foods of animal origin contain protein of high biological value. For this reason they may be important in African diets, which are often short of protein. But, unless produced by the family itself, such foods are usually too expensive for the average household, and are therefore not very frequently consumed. It is possible to have a balanced diet without meat or fish. The needed protein can come from cereals, legumes and other foods. Milk is important for infants and with eggs forms a useful addition to weaning diets.

Meat and meat products

Most adult Africans eat some kind of meat, depending on its availability and their incomes (see Fig. 52). The main values of meat in the diet are that it contains about 19 percent protein of excellent quality, and

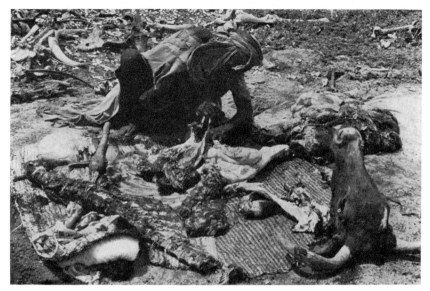

FIGURE 52. Dressing a carcass in the Niger.

iron that is well absorbed. The amount of fat depends on the animal that the meat comes from and the cut. The energy value of meat rises with the fat content. The fat is fairly high in its content of saturated fatty acids. Meat also provides useful amounts of riboflavin and niacin, a little thiamine, and small quantities of iron, vitamin A and vitamin C. Offal (the term used for the internal organs), and particularly liver, contains larger quantities. Offal has a relatively high amount of cholesterol.

The common belief that the white meat of birds is nutritionally superior to the red meat of land animals is untrue. In general the different groupings of animals — wild and domestic; large and small; birds, reptiles and mammals — all provide meat of similar nutritional value. The main variable is the fat content.

Under the heading of "meat" it seems appropriate to mention that in parts of Africa a wide range of animal products are eaten that are not generally eaten elsewhere. These include locusts and grasshoppers; termites, flying ants, lake flies, caterpillars, and other insects; baboons and monkeys; snakes and snails; rats and other rodents; and cats and dogs. The taste for these foods is no more strange than the French liking for frog's legs and snails and the English taste for eels and raw oysters. These foods are extremely nutritious, and contain protein of high biological value.

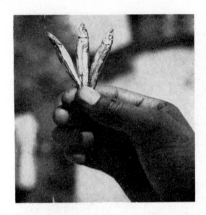

FIGURE 53. Dried *dagaa* are a rich source of calcium.

Fish

Fish, like meat, are valuable in the diet because they provide a good quantity (usually 17 percent or more) of protein of high biological value, particularly sulphur-containing amino acids. They are especially valuable as a complement to a cassava diet. Fish vary in their fat content but generally have less fat than meat. Fish also provide thiamine, riboflavin, niacin, vitamin A, iron and calcium. They contain a small quantity of vitamin C if eaten fresh.

Small fish, like sardines and sprats (*dagaa* in Tanzania, *kapenta* in Zambia) from the sea and lakes are consumed whole, bones and all, thus providing much calcium and fluorine (see Fig. 53). Dried *dagaa*, for instance, may contain 2 500 mg calcium/100 g.

Fish offal is not usually consumed. However, fish liver and fish oils are very rich sources of the fat-soluble vitamins A and D; the amount varies, usually with the age and species of fish.

Wherever water is available, fish provide a simple way of increasing protein consumption. The stocking of dams, the construction of fish ponds (see Fig. 54), better and more widespread fishing in rivers, lakes, or sea should all be given greater encouragement (see Fig. 55).

Although there is regional variation, it appears that African people will eat a greater variety of land animals than of sea creatures. Encouraging children in coastal districts to collect sea urchins, sea slugs, limpets and the numerous other edible sea creatures that abound, just as inland children collect locusts and lake flies, would considerably improve protein-poor diets. The introduction of swimming lessons in youth clubs and as a community development activity would develop this pastime as well as fishing both for pleasure and for profit. Fear of the water, because of inability to swim, is at present a deterrent to these activities.

186

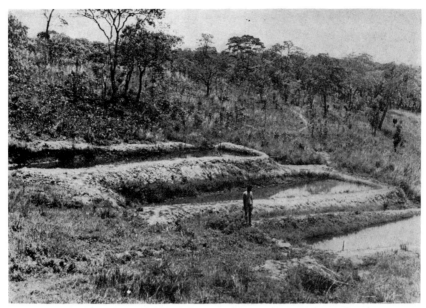

FIGURE 54. Construction of fish ponds should be encouraged wherever perennial water is available.

FIGURE 55. Fishing provides a useful spare-time activity for youngsters.

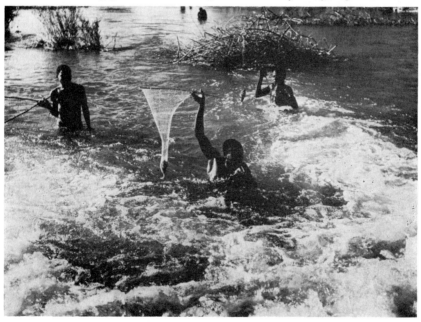

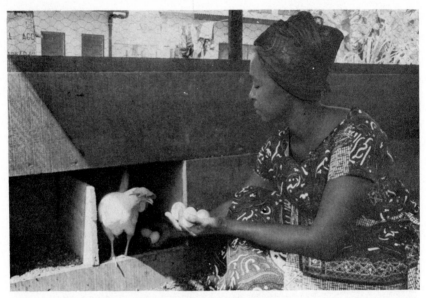

FIGURE 56. Backyard poultry-keeping in Accra, Ghana. Eggs provide an easily digestible, protein-rich food for infants and toddlers.

Eggs

The egg is one of the few foods containing no carbohydrate. Just as the foetus in its mother's uterus draws nutrients from its mother's blood in order that it may grow and develop into a human being, so the bird embryo draws all its nutrients from within the egg. It is not surprising therefore that eggs are highly nutritious. Egg contains a high proportion of excellent protein, is also rich in fat and contains good quantities of calcium and iron, vitamins A and D, and also thiamine and riboflavin.

Since eggs are an essential part of the reproductive cycle of birds, it is not surprising that many taboos forbid their consumption, particularly by women. It is gratifying that in many parts of Africa these taboos against eggs are fast disappearing, since the egg is one animal protein food universally available as a useful-sized unit. It is not often that a family can afford to kill a cow or even a goat for food, but eggs are small and frequently laid. They are also an easily prepared, easily digestible protein-rich food for children from the age of 6 months onward. Production of eggs for family use should be encouraged wherever possible (see Fig. 56), even in the small backyard of an urban dwelling. As a first priority, the eggs should be fed to the toddlers. Suitable methods of preparing eggs for children are mentioned in Chapter 36.

188

Blood

Cattle blood, which is regularly consumed by many pastoral peoples in Africa, is highly nutritious. It is rich in protein of high biological value and contains many other nutrients. It is a particularly valuable source of iron.

Milk and milk products

Milk is usually the only food consumed by an infant for the first few months of life. It forms a very important food for children, and can play a useful role in supplying missing nutrients in many adult diets.

The composition of milk varies with the animal it comes from, since the milk is designed for the rate of growth and other specific requirements of the young of that particular animal. Thus, for human infants, human breast milk is superior to cow's milk or any other milk product.

Except for certain vitamins previously mentioned, the composition of human breast milk remains fairly constant, regardless of the diet of the mother. A malnourished mother does not produce milk of markedly lower nutrient content, but instead reduces the quantity she is producing. The composition of human and cow's milk is compared below (adapted from Platt, 1962).

Milk	Carbohydrate (mainly lactose)	Protein	Fat	Calcium
	g/100 ml			*mg/100 ml*
Human	7.0	1.3	4.6	30
Cow's	4.7	3.3	3.6	120

Cow's milk contains the proteins caseinogen and lactalbumin. These proteins of high biological value are among its most important constituents (see Fig. 57). The carbohydrate present is the disaccharide lactose. The fat is present as very fine globules which, on standing, tend to coalesce and rise to the surface. The fat has a rather high content of saturated fatty acids. The calcium content of cow's milk (120 mg/100 ml) is four times that of human milk (30 mg/100 ml). This is one of nature's adaptations. It is because the calf grows much more quickly and has a larger

189

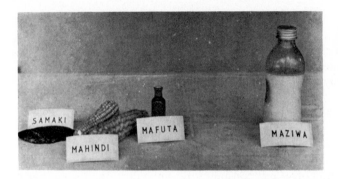

FIGURE 57. Milk *(maziwa)* contains protein present in fish *(samaki)*, fat present in oil *(mafuta)* and carbohydrate present in maize *(mahindi)*.

skeleton than the infant that it needs more calcium. When a human infant is fed entirely on cow's milk, the excess calcium causes no harm, nor does it affect the rate of growth beyond the optimum. The excess is excreted in the urine.

In addition to being an excellent source of protein of the best nutritive value, and of calcium, milk is a very good source of riboflavin and vitamin A. It is a fair source of thiamine and vitamin C, but it is a poor source of iron and niacin. The mother usually provides her infant with a store of iron before birth. However, this is exhausted by about the sixth month of life, and if prolonged feeding of milk alone takes place, iron deficiency anaemia may then develop.

The amount of thiamine in human milk varies more than the other constituents, and is largely dependent on the mother's intake of this vitamin. Infantile beriberi may occur in infants breast-fed by thiamine-deficient mothers. The vitamin A content of human milk is to some extent dependent on the diet of the mother.

Despite the variation in the composition of milk from different animals, all milk is rich in protein and other nutrients, and all constitute a good food for humans, especially children. If cow's milk is not available, then goats, sheep, or even camels should be milked. Some peoples have taboos against milk other than from a cow, and a few regard it as unsophisticated to drink goat's milk. From a nutritional point of view, this is unfortunate, since all these milks are valuable foods. In Scandinavia, even reindeer are milked.

In many parts of Africa, milk is more often consumed sour or curdled than fresh. There is no need to alter this habit — some tribes in fact dislike fresh milk — for curdled milk keeps longer, does not lose its nutritive value, and may be more digestible and more hygienic than fresh milk (see p. 18). However, it is very much safer to drink milk that has been boiled and kept in a clean container because milk can provide a vehicle for the transmission of some bacterial diseases.

190

Pasteurization of milk, if efficiently carried out in a large, well-run dairy and provided that milk is placed in clean containers destined for direct delivery to the consumer, will reduce greatly the risk of spread of pathological organisms. However, in many small towns where so-called pasteurization is not well controlled, the milk may be insufficiently heated, the containers may not be well cleaned, and the milk may go from the plant into large churns for bottling elsewhere in unsanitary surroundings. The consumer should not be over-confident in all milk labelled "pasteurized", since it is not necessarily free from pathological organisms.

In many countries where cow's milk is a normal item of the diet, it is customary to wean the infant from the mother's breast milk onto a diet of which cow's milk forms an important part (see Fig. 58). This is a valuable practice for it then helps ensure that the child will receive a balanced diet providing all the requirements for growth, development and health.

In recent years there has been some concern about the condition known as lactose intolerance, which has been found in some non-white people. This is not likely to cause problems among Africans accustomed to drinking milk in moderate quantities.

Skim milk and dried skim milk. Skim milk is milk from which the fat has been removed, usually for making butter. In its dried form (DSM), it is a familiar product in many African countries. It contains nearly all the milk protein, as well as the carbohydrate, calcium and B vitamins. It is an excellent food, especially for those on predominantly carbohydrate

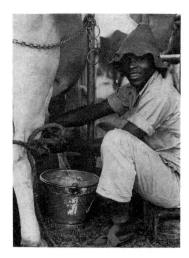

FIGURE 58. Milking time at Egerton College of Agriculture, Njoro, Kenya. Better cattle, better managed, provide more and richer milk.

diets, and for those who have extra needs for protein (but see footnote on p. 103). For the latter, i.e., the young child, the pregnant woman and the lactating mother, skim milk is in some places supplied at clinics and health centres to those in special need. It is extensively used in hospitals and dispensaries as the basis for the curative treatment of protein-energy malnutrition (see p. 119). It is also issued at child-welfare clinics to prevent this most devastating form of malnutrition. Skim milk is an excellent food to add to or supplement any diet, but it is particularly useful in those of children and pregnant and lactating women. However, it is not a suitable substitute for whole milk for an infant. It is sometimes added to dietary supplements such as, for example, CSM (corn/soya/milk mixture).

Whole powdered milk. This, as the name implies, is whole milk that has been dried. Unlike DSM, it contains also the fat. It is suitable for infants when no breast milk is available.

Evaporated and condensed milks. These are milks from which much of the water has been removed but which are still liquid. Condensed milk is sweetened by the addition of sugar, while evaporated milk does not contain added sugar. Many brands of condensed milk have vitamins added. These brands should be used in preference to those which do not have vitamins added especially if used in the diet of young children. Evaporated whole milk is suitable for infants but evaporated skim milk and condensed milks should not be fed to infants in place of breast milk or whole milk.

Yoghurt and soured or fermented milks. As mentioned, many Africans prefer soured milk to fresh milk. A wide variety of organisms are used in the process of making yoghurt and fermented milks. These products are easy to prepare, are highly nutritious, have enhanced keeping quality and are a little less likely to harbour pathogenic organisms than is fresh milk. Their use should be encouraged.

Casein. This is the protein part of the milk. It tends to be rather expensive and is sold under various proprietary names (e.g., "Casilan-Glaxo"). It is commonly mixed as part of a "formula" or mixture for treatment of children with protein-energy malnutrition (see p. 120). It is a relatively expensive product.

Butter and ghee. These are both milk products, but since they are mainly fat they are discussed below under "Oils and fats".

192

Cheese. The making of cheese no doubt arose out of the desire of farm people to preserve some of the excess milk of the summer. Numerous processes are used, but essentially cheese is made by letting milk clot and subsequently removing some of the water. Salt and other flavourings may be added. Cheese is not widely eaten by rural Africans. However, attempts are being made to popularize it, for there is no doubt that, in cattle country, cheese making would be an excellent way of using any excess milk produced during the wet season.

28. OILS AND FATS

A diet very low in fat tends to be unpalatable and dull. Fats, however, like proteins, are relatively expensive, and so the diet of poorer people is often short of fat. Fat is important because it provides, weight for weight, more than twice as much energy as carbohydrate or protein, thus reducing the bulk of the diet. Fats and oils may be good sources of fat-soluble vitamins, and assist with the absorption of other nutrients. Recent work has established that certain unsaturated fatty acids are essential for health. But above all, it is difficult to cook a really good meal without any fat or oil, although the desired amount is largely a matter of habit and taste.

Fats contain a variety of fatty acids. Those derived from land animals usually contain a high proportion of saturated fatty acids and are solid at room temperature (e.g., butter, lard). Fats derived from vegetable products and marine animals contain more unsaturated fatty acids; they are usually liquid at room temperature (e.g., groundnut oil, cod-liver oil) and are termed oils. Coconut oil is an exception in that it contains mainly saturated fatty acids. A high intake of saturated fatty acids may contribute to raised serum cholesterol levels, which in turn may increase the risk of coronary heart disease.

Butter

Butter consists mainly of the fat from milk. It usually contains about 82 percent fat, with a trace of protein and carbohydrate; the rest is water. Butter is rich in vitamin A and has a small amount of vitamin D, but the content varies with the time of year, and the diet of the cow from which it was derived. Usually about 3 000 IU of vitamin A[1] and 50 IU

---

[1] Comprising 640 µg retinol plus 545 µg β-carotene equivalent.

of vitamin D are present in 100 g. Butter is becoming popular in African diets with the increased use of bread.

Margarine

This has been developed as a substitute for butter. It is made from a variety of vegetable oils that are partially hydrogenated to give a product with a consistency similar to butter. In most countries vitamins A and D are added so that the final product is nutritionally very similar to butter. If these vitamins have been added, it will usually say so on the margarine container.

Ghee

Ghee is made by boiling milk fat to precipitate the protein which is then removed. It contains 99 percent fat, no protein or carbohydrate, about 2 000 IU of vitamin A [1]/100 g and some vitamin D. It has good keeping qualities and is much used in tropical countries in place of butter, since the latter soon goes rancid if kept unrefrigerated in warm climates.

Lard

Lard is collected during the heating of pork. Like other similar animal fats (e.g., dripping, suet), it consists of 99 percent fat and contains no carbohydrate, proteins, vitamins, or minerals.

Vegetable oils

These are the cooking fats most commonly used in Africa, and a large variety exists. Except for red palm oil, they have the disadvantage, compared with some of the previously mentioned fats, that they contain no vitamins. They are mainly low in their content of saturated fatty acids.

Commonly used vegetable oils are groundnut oil, sunflower oil, sesame oil, cottonseed oil, and coconut oil. In their pure form, they are 100 percent fat and contain no water or other nutrients. A large number of proprietary preparations are available, of which "Kimbo" is the best known in East Africa. Red palm oil is widely produced in West Africa,

---

[1] Comprising 420 µg retinol plus 360 µg β-carotene equivalent.

but not much in East Africa. The oil contains large quantities of carotene, the precursor of vitamin A, commonly 12 000 µg [with a range from 600 to 60 000 µg/100 g (Platt, 1962)]. It is therefore a very valuable food wherever a shortage of vitamin A occurs in the diet. Red palm oil should thus be the fat used in all institutional diets in Africa, for it is not much more expensive than other oils. Vitamin A deficiency will not be a problem in areas where all members of the family consume even small quantities of red palm oil. Encouragement should be given to its wider cultivation and consumption in East Africa and areas to the south.

29. BEVERAGES AND CONDIMENTS

Beverages

It is essential that the human body receive water, yet the human taste prefers that much of this water be obtained in the form of beverages. These include beer, wine, spirits, fruit juices, tea, coffee, cocoa, synthetic sweetened soft drinks, and aerated waters. Some of these contain small amounts of drugs such as caffeine (tea, coffee and some colas), or alcohol in varying amounts (beer, wine and spirits), and some are sources of minerals and vitamins.

In Africa many beverages are made from cereal grains after the grain has been soaked and has sprouted. This enhances the nutritive value and these beverages, if consumed without filtration or distillation, often contain good quantities of B vitamins. A few of these beverages such as *togwa* in East Africa are non-alcoholic. Some have a high energy content and a fair amount of protein.

Fruit juices made in the home from fresh fruit are usually rich sources of vitamin C, and some contain carotene. Only the highest grade of fruit squashes and practically none of the bottled, aerated fruit drinks or sodas have any vitamins. None contain anywhere near the vitamin content of fresh fruit juice. Yet it is not uncommon to find mothers giving their babies and children orange squash or fruit-flavoured sodas because they were told at the clinic to give them fruit juice. This will do no good to the child and is a waste of money. These sugar-sweetened soft drinks and sodas may also be a contributing cause of dental caries (tooth decay).

There are, however, certain vitamin-rich proprietary beverages designed for infants and children. The vitamin content of these is nearly always clearly stated on the label. Such beverages are not necessary if the child is getting fresh fruit and vegetables. They are often a very expensive way of providing vitamin C to a child, despite the advertising that tends to persuade the mother otherwise.

Some natural waters from rivers, lakes, wells, or springs are good sources of calcium, magnesium or fluoride.

Condiments

Salt consists mainly of sodium chloride. It is the only mineral salt that man customarily consumes in a chemically pure form. The body has a definite need for sodium and chlorine. The amount of sodium chloride in the body is regulated by the kidneys. In hot countries a person doing heavy work may lose 15 g of sodium chloride in body sweat in one day. Urinary excretion ranges from 1 g to 30 g or more per day. Despite this loss, except where sweating is profuse, salt is not essential in man's diet, since sufficient sodium and chlorine can be obtained from food alone. Nevertheless, salt is a commodity that nearly every person, however little money he has, will buy if he cannot dig it or make it himself. Adults usually consume about 10 g of salt a day, but there are enormous variations. Certainly a salt-free diet is a most unpalatable one, but possibly this is because our palates have been educated to like a salty taste from a very early age. A high intake of salt may contribute to the development of hypertension or high blood pressure.

Others spices and flavourings are of less physiological or nutritive importance. In all countries, in all ages, man has added such items to his food to improve and to vary its taste. Few of these have much nutritional importance. In Africa a variety of wild leaves is used, partly for flavour, partly as vegetable *per se*; hot chilies, both red and green, are frequently used; pepper and curry powder are popular additions to the sauce or stew accompanying the staple. Some have nutritive value, some do not, but all serve to make the food more pleasing to the taste, and they therefore both increase the appetite and assist digestion by stimulating the secretion of saliva and intestinal juices. With the march of so-called civilization, many of the traditional and natural condiments and herbs are being replaced by proprietary sauces and flavourings. Some of these are artificial chemical agents, and some are based on traditional spices.

V. NUTRITION POLICY AND PROGRAMMES

30. FOOD AND NUTRITION POLICY

General problems of poverty and deprivation [1]

Many parts of Africa have in recent years experienced an acute food crisis and some have suffered from serious famine. All the countries of Africa have major problems of malnutrition in certain sectors of their populations. That these problems have persisted, and in some cases worsened despite an increased pace of development, is due to many and diverse factors. These include adverse weather, the spiralling costs of fuel and fertilizer while prices of African export commodities dropped or failed to keep pace, and a grave shortage of foreign exchange.

Undernutrition and malnutrition are an important part of the complex, widespread problem of poverty and deprivation that affects millions, perhaps the majority, of people in Africa. The poor, the hungry and the malnourished are unable to live a normal life, they are less likely to fulfil their potential as human beings, and they cannot contribute fully to the development of their own countries. The numbers of persons who are poor or malnourished or both appear to be increasing in many countries. This is, in part, because the population of many nations is increasing more rapidly than are the services and goods necessary to relieve malnutrition and poverty. But it is also clear that economic gains as assured by gross national product or industrial output are not reflected in improvements in the quality of life of the majority of ordinary people. Often the gap between the rich and the poor is widening.

Malnutrition and infections combine to pose an enormous hazard to the health of the majority of the world's population who live in poverty. This ever-present threat applies particularly to children under 5 years old. Many of the children who suffer from both malnutrition and a series of

---

[1] This section is adapted from Latham, 1975.

infections succumb and die. They are continually replaced by parents who have a strong desire, and often a real need, to have surviving children. The children who live beyond 5 years of age are not mainly those who have escaped malnutrition or infectious diseases, but those who have survived. They are seldom left without the permanent sequelae or scars of their early health experiences. They are often retarded in their physical, psychological, or behavioural development, and they may have other abnormalities that may contribute to a reduced ability to function optimally as adults and possibly to a shortened life expectation. Other factors influencing the development of these children include a lack of environmental stimulation and a host of deprivations related to poverty.

The challenge to health workers and to development economists, to governments and to international agencies is how best to reduce the morbidity, mortality, and permanent sequelae that result from this synergism of malnutrition and infection. The answer is not sophisticated hospitals such as those erected in the capital cities and provincial centres of developing countries, and it does not lie in elaborate manufactured foods such as spun soy protein or expensive infant formulas. Neither is there need for more highly trained doctors or for advanced food technology. To tackle this huge problem the affluent nations should resolve to make the reduction of deprivation a primary goal, and the governments of African countries should also accept this as a priority.

Objectives of development. The governments in both the developed and developing countries must first decide what "development" really means. Too often in the past, development has been viewed mainly in terms of industrialization, and measured in terms of productive capacity and material output of a country. Indicators of development were GNP or mean per caput incomes.

Economists have tended to view improved nutrition and health as welfare questions. But it is now clear that these classical patterns of development often contribute very little to the quality of life of the majority of citizens of any country, and may sometimes aggravate the problems of the poor. We need therefore to ask, What is the purpose of economic development? Who is it for? If improved health and better nutrition for people are not considered in development plans, then one might seriously question whether this really is development.

Developing countries should, of course, strive for overall economic development, and especially for improvements in agricultural development. Support, however, should be given largely to those projects and that type of development that will benefit a large segment of the population, will help reduce inequalities in income distribution, and are likely to improve the nutrition, health, and quality of life of those currently deprived. For

198

example, labour-intensive projects are often preferable to capital-intensive ones, and support for small farmers to that for large estates.

The control of infectious diseases and projects aimed at providing more and better food for people are fully justified and important components of a development plan. By themselves they may contribute to increased productivity and better lives. An improved infant or toddler mortality rate, a lowered disease incidence, and a better nourished population are perhaps better indicators of development than national averages of telephones or automobiles per thousand families, or even than per caput income. For example, who would claim that development is far behind in China when childhood malnutrition has apparently been almost eliminated, major communicable diseases controlled, and the population increase stabilized? Yet China has very many fewer private telephones or automobiles per family and a much lower per caput income than many countries where malnutrition is common, health is poor, and the population is rising rapidly.

It is not possible here to provide a blue-print for development that includes the objectives of reducing infectious diseases and improving food intake. However, it is increasingly being realized that primary health care can be effectively delivered by persons with considerably less training than doctors, and that there are advantages in having many auxiliary medical workers in widely scattered dispensaries and health centres in villages and rural areas rather than having a few doctors and a hierarchy of supporting staff in hospitals in the principal towns. Most common illnesses can be successfully treated by health auxiliaries with simple equipment and a limited range of medicines. A health system using auxiliaries can be devised to place much more emphasis on preventive rather than curative medicine. Auxiliaries can give immunizations, provide maternal and child-health services including family planning, administer simple nutrition programmes, and direct local public-health measures.

Satisfying energy needs. It is now also widely accepted that most of the malnutrition in developing countries is due to inadequate intake of food, and is often associated with infectious diseases. Protein deficiency is not the most important nutrition problem in the world. There has been an over-emphasis on the protein problem and too much stress on protein deficiencies with a relative neglect of the first goal of a good policy, which should be to satisfy the energy needs of the population. In most populations where the staple food is a cereal such as rice, wheat, maize or millet, serious protein deficiencies seldom occur except where there is also an energy or overall food deficiency. Most cereals contain 8-12 percent protein and are often consumed with moderate quantities of legumes and vegetables. If energy requirements are met on these diets, protein deficiencies usually become rare, and are certainly confined mainly to very young children suffering increased nitrogen losses due to frequent infections. However, among those whose staple is plantain, cassava, or some other food with a low protein content, the situation may be very different.

The lesson to be learned is that commercial production of relatively expensive protein-rich foods, the amino-acid fortification of cereal grains, the production of single-cell protein, and several other ventures that a few years ago were offered as panaceas for the world's nutrition problems can only reduce the problem of protein-energy malnutrition by a very small degree. Similarly, attempts at making small changes in the amino-acid pattern of cereal grains by means of genetic manipulation are much less important than increasing the yields per hectare of these cereals, and of other food crops. Of far greater importance are measures that would enable people to purchase the foods they need.

A modest increase in cereal, legume and vegetable consumption by children will greatly reduce the prevalence of protein-energy malnutrition and growth deficits of children in Africa, especially if combined with control of infectious diseases. Breast-feeding during the first few months of life can assure an adequate diet, whereas bottle-feeding is a major cause of diarrhoea and nutritional marasmus.

Other prophylactic programmes. Fairly simple and relatively inexpensive nutrition programmes can be used to control specific nutritional problems, the most important of which are vitamin A deficiency, which is a major cause of blindness; iodine deficiency which leads to goitre and endemic cretinism; and iron or folate deficiency, which leads to anaemias. For example, in some areas xerophthalmia is being controlled by providing all young children with a capsule containing 60 000 µg retinol (200 000 IU of vitamin A) every 6 months; in other areas this is done by fortifying commonly eaten foods with the vitamin. Vitamin A is a relatively inexpensive nutrient *per se*; the major cost is in the delivery system. There is no reason why blindness due to vitamin A deficiency cannot be almost totally eliminated everywhere within the next 10 years. Mandatory iodization of salt has been remarkably successful in reducing goitre and mental deficiency associated with cretinism in several countries. Nutritional anaemias could be controlled by using similar simple methods.

Synergistic services. The control of infectious diseases and the improvement of nutrition both deserve a high priority in development plans and in international or bilateral assistance to African countries. They should be instituted together because they will be mutually reinforcing and cost less if provided in a coordinated manner rather than separately. Historical and epidemiological evidence suggests that reduction in infant and child mortality and improvement in health and nutritional status may be pre-requisites to successful family-spacing efforts. In the over-populated countries of the world, population control deserves high priority, and parents in all countries should receive assistance to help them achieve their desired family size.

It seems logical to recommend coordinated programmes that have three objectives, namely, to control infectious disease, to improve nutrition, and to make family-planning services widely available. These three types of services may together be synergistic.

National food and nutrition policy

Food and nutrition policies should be an integrated and important part of national development plans. However, although included in past 5-year development plans in Tanzania and Zambia, for example, they have been given insufficient attention in most African countries.

The general objectives of a food and nutrition policy will be to improve the quantity and quality of food eaten by the population, with the aim of ensuring an adequate diet for all people. In nutrition there exists the paradox that overconsumption of food or of certain dietary items also carries a risk to health. For example, consumption of food above the needs for energy expenditure leads to obesity, and the high intakes of cholesterol and saturated fats typical in western diets that are high in animal products increase the risk of heart disease. A more equitable distribution of food between the poor and the affluent might thus improve the health of both groups.

The implications of a national food and nutrition policy should cover the following three different areas: food supply, food demand and biological utilization.

Food supply. If a population is to be adequately nourished then there must be an adequate quantity of food in the country of the right quality. Therefore a fundamental strategy of a food policy must be to improve and increase food production. How this should be achieved is mainly an agricultural question. However, decision makers in agriculture need to be made aware of the nutritional needs of the population, to understand the nutritional implications of their actions, and to appreciate that agricultural policy affects food prices, which in turn affect food consumption. In general in Africa there is a need to expand the production of certain foodstuffs, especially those cereals and legumes currently eaten in a given area. Where livestock such as cattle are competing with man for food or for agriculturally productive land it is preferable, from a nutritional point of view, to give priority to the cultivation of cereals, legumes, root crops and vegetables, rather than animals. Similarly a greater concentration on food crops rather than cash crops is generally desirable.

A second aspect of food supply is that of food marketing, including transport and storage. It should be part of policy to make this logical, as simple as possible, well-organized, and with a minimum involvement of middlemen. This will help to ensure that the producer gets a fair return for his produce and that the consumer pays the lowest reasonable price for his food. Cooperatives are one form of marketing that may benefit both producer and consumer.

Other factors besides food production and marketing that affect food supply are commercial food processing and industrialization, and the policies related to importation and exportation of food, that is, including food donated in multilateral or bilateral agreements.

Food demand. This is largely determined by per caput incomes and by food prices. Since the poor are the most vulnerable to food deficits and malnutrition, any policies that increase their purchasing power will provide them with the potential to improve their nutrition. Therefore increased employment and better wages become components of a nutrition policy. In many African countries the minority of the working population are employed in the sense of receiving wages. Most are self-employed in agriculture. Assistance to this group of poor farmers to increase their incomes and their food productivity will have a similar effect to increasing the wages of the urban poor.

Allied to employment and income policy will be government tax policies, which should ensure a fair distribution of wealth if the objective of improving the nutrition of the poor is to be realized.

Food prices affect both supply and demand. If prices are low the farmer generally gets little for his produce and if too low he has little desire to produce or to sell. However, lower prices represent an increase in the purchasing power of the consumer. A lowering of the price of a common staple food such as maize meal is equivalent to raising the incomes or spending capacity of all those who purchase this food. Similarly, raising the price (a more common occurrence) is equivalent to lowering the income of those who purchase it. Governments have various mechanisms at their disposal to help satisfy the needs of both producers and consumers. One of these is to subsidize the price of a food, i.e., to increase the price paid to the farmer for a bag of maize without increasing the price that the consumer has to pay for it in the market or shop. This may be costly for the government but it may help the poor to improve their nutrition. Too often in the past pricing policies and subsidies have been directed at foods consumed mainly by the high-income groups. For

202

example, a price restriction on cheese or powdered milk or tinned baby foods, or a subsidy on beef or margarine would hardly benefit the poor at all, and would have little or no nutritional impact. This would be so even if the poor were for example short of protein, and could benefit nutritionally from an increased consumption of meat.

Other policies that affect demand and that can be used to improve the nutrition of poor families include supplementary feeding, nutrition education, consumer guidance and family-spacing.

Biological utilization. This third area of policy is seldom considered by economists, but it tends to be the major area of concern to health workers and even nutritionists. Its implications are discussed elsewhere in this manual. Its elements include the control of infectious and parasitic diseases that are strongly related to malnutrition; attention to ecological factors related to health and nutrition; the increase and improvement of health services, especially simple services available to the poor; food cleanliness and hygiene; domestic water supplies and environmental sanitation; child-spacing; and health and nutrition education.

In the past many government measures have in fact unwittingly aggravated and increased malnutrition because the nutritional implications of the policy had not been considered. Examples of measures that have increased malnutrition include: price and wage regulations, tax policies, over-attention to cash-crop rather than food-crop production, diversion of a major share of the health budget to national and regional hospitals rather than to rural health units and preventive health services. Even specific nutrition programmes have been doomed to failure because they never reach the families of the poor or the most vulnerable groups. Examples of this include some programmes to manufacture and sell protein-rich weaning foods, nutrition education that encourages mothers to feed meat and eggs to their children every day, subsidized school lunches in fee-paying secondary schools, amino-acid enrichment of a cereal when the amino acid used may be limiting in that cereal but not in the diets of the malnourished poor, and subsidizing of milk production.

31. GOVERNMENT ORGANIZATION
FOR NUTRITION POLICY AND PLANNING

The need for coordination of nutrition policy and planning has already been stressed. The main nutrition activities will be undertaken by government departments and ministries because nearly all African countries are governed under a system that divides the functions of government in this way. Therefore, unless a separate ministry of food and nutrition is established, there needs to be some other mechanism to ensure the proper planning and coordination of a national food and nutrition policy. The objective is to ensure that the components of the nutrition policy within the various ministries are fully compatible, coordinated and, if possible, harmonized. The implementation of programmes, however, should remain with the existing ministries, departments and agencies.

At present, ministries are in dialogue with both the overall political authority of the country and also with a central planning body responsible for overall development plans and for the budget of the various government ministries.

Certain ministries will have responsibility for particular aspects of programme implementation, or for certain nutrition programmes in which the ministries of health, agriculture and education should be particularly involved. The ministries responsible for local government, rural development and social services or community development will also play an important role. In many African countries various institutions or committees have been established to provide for the coordination of nutrition activities. In Zambia a national food and nutrition commission was set up soon after independence. The Tanzanian Food and Nutrition Centre has been established as a parastatal body with responsibility to the Ministry of Health in Tanzania. In many other countries there are interministerial committees to discuss nutrition matters that concern several ministries.

Generally there exists no unit or organization that identifies, appraises and recommends in a systematic and comprehensive manner the measures and strategies that a government might use to meet the objectives of an adequate diet for the population. Similarly there is seldom a structure or unit that analyses the nutritional implications of the development plan and of other programmes of government ministries. There is clearly a need to provide the function of overview.

The Joint FAO/WHO Expert Committee on Nutrition (FAO, 1976) states that:

> Responsibility, capability, and authority for overview need to be assigned to a body so placed that it can affect the decisions of the planning authority (ministry of planning, central planning body) with regard to the programmes and budgets of the ministries.
> In practice, such a planning body (let us call it a food and nutrition planning unit) should be in a position to require the various ministries to join a dialogue and provide information on the nutritional impact and costs of their activities. It needs a capacity for independent analysis and it is further desirable that it should have the capacity to

assist the ministries — singly or together — to identify, design and appraise programmes. One of its major roles, too, will be to assist the ministries to build their own planning capacities and effective decision-making machinery by, for example, developing appraisal and design criteria for programmes and projects. In practice, this also means that the unit should be financially independent of the operating ministries and act on sufficiently high authority for it to be taken seriously both within the ministries and at higher policy-making levels.

The food and nutrition planning unit should seek to secure a shared view of the nature of the nutrition problem, overall and in its various aspects and local manifestations, and a shared understanding of the role that each ministry is to play in the overall process of nutrition planning and in the coordination of implementation. For these reasons, it will, from time to time, be desirable to convene working groups attended by members of the various ministries which might also consider, on an *ad hoc* basis, specific components of food and nutrition policy. They might also bring in, as appropriate, people from other agencies — nutrition institutes, universities, etc.

The food and nutrition planning unit would need to have its own technical expertise and analytical capacity, but it may need also to draw on technical support groups in such fields as nutrition, public health, economics and agricultural economics, statistics, education and extension, management, and marketing.

The food and nutrition planning unit would report to the body responsible for overall inter-ministry coordination and national development policy making. It would prepare the briefings that ensure that sectoral plans come under scrutiny for their impact on the overall national nutrition situation. The composite of policies and programmes resulting from this process will be the national food and nutrition strategy. To some extent, this might be reflected in the preparation of a food and nutrition plan document, which might also be the responsibility of the unit, but this is not the essential feature of effective food and nutrition planning.

The author was a member of the above Joint FAO/WHO Expert Committee on Nutrition and believes that such a unit (commission, centre of whatever it is termed) could with great advantage be established in most African countries. In Zambia and in Tanzania this might mean the strengthening and redrafting of the terms of reference of the present Commission and Centre respectively. In other countries it might entail the establishment of a new unit, as is planned in Kenya, perhaps under the Ministry of Finance and Planning or in the President's office.

Food and nutrition policy is too important a part of national development to be ignored or to be dealt with broken down as completely separate components of the activities of several ministries. All those concerned with nutrition can play a role, first by coordinating their activities with those of colleagues in other ministries and secondly by influencing the government to establish a suitable nutrition policy, planning and coordination unit in his or her country.

But beyond the need for national cooperation of ministries and departments, cooperation is vital at a district and village level if plans to improve nutrition are to be really effective. There are different committees and bodies that form suitable venues for formulating cooperative ideas. This may in one country be the district team, in another a district development committee, in a third a locally formed Freedom From Hunger committee. A body such as any of these, with the senior administrative or political figure as chairman, and with representatives drawn from the different ministries, can agree on a coordinated policy to improve nutrition, and then take action. A doctor can investigate and report on medical problems. An agricultural officer and his veterinary colleagues can then outline how best to solve the problem within the existing pattern of agriculture. An education officer and community development officer can assist by educating people to improve their own conditions.

In the village a similar committee in miniature can implement plans in the same spirit of cooperation. The committee responsible might again be the village development committee, or it might be a committee specially formed to improve nutrition. This committee might consist of the local political leaders and village headmen, the schoolteacher, the medical assistant or rural medical aide, the agricultural and veterinary field officers, the community development assistants, the chairman of the local cooperative society, and other suitable persons such as a traditional healer and traditional midwife.

The following example illustrates how this type of cooperative effort might work in practice.

Example. The district medical officer, having conducted a small clinical survey, would inform the district team of his findings. The main problem discovered might be protein deficiency resulting from a diet predominantly of cassava. The agricultural officer might advise that though most of the land is unsuitable for maize, nevertheless millet would grow, that legume production could be increased and that it would be feasible to build fishponds and to increase poultry raising.

The local village committee could, on its own initiative or after instruction from the district headquarters, decide on how to take action. It might be decided first to tackle the problem where it existed. The medical assistant would prepare a record of all families in which protein-energy malnutrition had occurred. The households would be visited by him or a health nurse. Information about the diet would be obtained and advice given, especially about foods for young children.

The agricultural field officer would inspect the farm or *shamba*. He might advise on where an extra hectare of millet could best be planted, and suggest that maize could be grown in the valley bottom in rotation with beans. He would agree to exchange a good cockerel for the local poor one. He might further choose a site and give advice regarding construction of a fishpond. The community development assistant would follow to give advice regarding the right food for young children. He would demonstrate the addition of beans and an occasional egg to gruel for the toddler. The cooperative assistant might arrange that a retail cooperative shop be started. The political leader might find that fertile areas of land were not being cultivated because of archaic land inheritance laws based on old traditions. He could arrange for better land usage.

All this might be done in a village by a team of people working together. There are also community activities that can be performed on a self-help or "nation-building" basis that will improve nutrition. An enlightened village committee could try to see that every household planted a certain quota of fruit trees, grew a certain area of legumes, kept poultry for its own use, and so on. It might prefer to start a communal orchard near the village source of water. It might build below this a large village fishpond, or it might introduce a midday meal in the village school. Measures to improve nutrition will thus vary from country to country, area to area, village to village.

32. NUTRITION PROGRAMMES AND HEALTH STRATEGIES

Food shortages, low incomes, land pressure and deprivations are among the many root causes of malnutrition. The elimination of these common African problems will take time, resourcefulness, money and political resolve. While governments begin to tackle these monstrous problems the extent of malnutrition can be lessened by a number of nutrition programmes and health strategies. These are not alternative approaches but should be coordinated efforts that proceed simultaneously. Thus, while the government grapples with the problems of poverty and deprivation, some direct intervention programmes aimed specifically at improving nutrition can be implemented.

Suggestions for measures aimed at the prevention of each important deficiency disease are included at the end of the chapter describing that particular form of malnutrition. Discussion here will focus on four more general measures that have not been covered adequately elsewhere. These are: food fortification or enrichment, supplementary foods, medicinal nutrients, and nutrition education. Other equally important general measures are the control of infectious diseases (Chapter 1), family-spacing (Chapter 3) and child-health services (Chapter 19).

Food fortification or enrichment

The term fortification is used here for the addition of one or more nutrients to a food for the purpose of improving its nutritional value. This method has proved very successful for the control of certain forms of malnutrition. The advantages of fortification are that it can improve the nutritional status of people without any special action or change of behaviour on their part and that it is usually fairly inexpensive.

The difficulties and disadvantages of fortification are several. It is necessary to find a food suitable for fortification; one that passes through a limited number of manufacturing or processing plants where a nutrient can be added, and is consumed at regular intervals by the nutritionally vulnerable groups of the population. Conditions are unsuitable for fortification if the amount of the proposed food consumed varies very widely and if the nutrient to be added is toxic in large amounts or changes the quality of the food, including its taste and colour, and if the usual preparation and cooking of the food cause deterioration in the nutrient to be added.

Fortification is only desirable if the deficiency to be corrected is fairly prevalent or the nutrient to be added is very cheap. Ideally, the addition of the nutrient should not cause any marked increase in the cost of the food to the consumer. Clearly, any addition will add to the cost but this may be borne either by the government or the manufacturer, or by a very modest rise in the price of the commodity. In most instances it is desirable that government legislation be enacted to make mandatory the fortification of a particular food or group of foods with specified levels of particular nutrients. It is then essential to have a good system of control and supervision to ensure that manufacturers are abiding by the legislation.

The best example of a successful fortification programme is one in which iodine is added to salt as a means of preventing endemic goitre. This has been practised in many countries, both industrialized and developing, for several decades. For example, Colombia has had legislation for the iodization of salt for over 20 years. In the province of Caldas, the goitre rate was about 80 percent prior to iodization, around 10 percent 3 years later and was down to less than 2 percent after 10 years. The fortification of salt with iodine has been among the nutrition success stories. Salt, as a vehicle for fortification, has many advantages over other foods. The amount consumed does not vary widely, it is almost universally purchased and consumed, and in many countries there are only a limited number of producers.

The addition of fluoride to water supplies has proved of definite benefit in the control of dental caries (tooth decay). Fluoride will not totally prevent dental caries but if taken in specified amounts during childhood will very greatly reduce the amount of dental caries and the number of teeth lost. Fluoridation is only possible where there is a good piped-water supply and where the amount of fluoride added can be controlled. Cereal flours in many countries have been fortified with B vitamins. This is a useful procedure where deficiencies of these vitamins are common, where a suitable cereal flour is widely consumed by those at risk, and where most of the milling is done by large concerns capable of properly fortifying these products. Recently attempts have been made to control xerophthalmia by the addition of vitamin A to a number of foodstuffs. These include sugar, salt, tea and monosodium glutamate (a flavouring widely used in Asia). The feasibility and effectiveness of these measures are being evaluated. Vitamin A has for years been added to foods such as margarine in the industrialized countries, and is being added to dried skim milk used in food aid, as previously mentioned.

Nutritional anaemias are a widespread problem in many countries. The fortification of a suitable foodstuff with iron and possibly also with folate offers the possibility of an easy control measure. To date, attempts have been limited by technological and other problems.

Another use for fortification may be to replace nutrients that are lost in processing, or that may be present in the natural food for which the manufactured food is a substitute. Margarine enriched with vitamin A as a butter substitute, and highly milled cereals enriched with B vitamins replacing lightly milled or home-pounded cereals are examples already cited. The addition of vitamin A and other nutrients to breast-milk substitutes, and vitamin C to fruit-based bottled drinks provide other examples.

In general, when a specific nutritional deficiency exists in a country or part of a country, consideration should be given to the feasibility of controlling the condition using a fortification programme, since this may well be the cheapest and most effective available means of control.

Medicinal nutrients

The provision of specific nutrients in medicinal form to groups of the population is another way to control malnutrition. All the vitamin and mineral nutrients can be used in this way. Any nutrient that is suitable for fortification could as an alternative be given medicinally to groups of the population.

The disadvantage of this method compared with fortification is that the delivery system is of necessity more difficult and much more expensive. When medicinal nutrients are provided in a control programme it is impossible to reach all those in need, and it is often the most vulnerable people who are the most difficult to reach. The advantage is that the nutrient can be selectively administered to those at risk whereas with fortification many well-nourished persons not requiring additional quantities of the nutrient receive it.

The provision of iron tablets to pregnant women attending antenatal or prenatal clinics has been successfully practised in many countries for a long time. It is a good means of reducing the risk of iron deficiency anaemia during pregnancy. In Africa most women do not attend clinics during their pregnancies, and those who do attend are often the affluent and educated. Nevertheless, the practice of providing iron is a valuable one and should be continued; at the same time, increased attendance should be encouraged at these clinics and more of them should be established in remote areas.

Fluoride tablets taken by children on a regular basis are an effective way of limiting dental caries in areas where the local water supply is low in fluoride (containing less than 0.5 parts per million).

The provision of high-dose capsules of vitamin A to children every 4 or 6 months as a means of preventing xerophthalmia is being increasingly practised. In some countries niacin tablets to prevent pellagra are regularly issued in certain institutions.

Such programmes are to be recommended wherever there is a need. However, most of the vitamin and mineral pills manufactured and sold throughout the world are taken by persons who are adequately nourished and have no need for the additional nutrients. On the whole, most unnecessary pill-taking does no harm to health, but it is a waste of the consumer's money. In a few cases the excessive use of these pills, especially those rich in vitamins A and D, may cause toxicity and occasionally serious illness.

Supplementary foods and feeding programmes

Two aspects of supplementary foods merit consideration. The first is to determine the need for them in a particular country or area, and the second, to decide whether a feeding programme should be established.

It is generally recognized that the weaning period is a critical one from a nutritional point of view. Breast milk alone is adequate for the first 4 to 6 months, and then while breast-feeding continues other foods need to be introduced. Thus, there is a period between about 5 months of age and up to about 3 years of age during which the infant or young child needs more than breast milk but cannot do well on the limited number of meals and the type of food that older members of the family may be consuming.

As mentioned in Part VI, there are many excellent traditional ways of feeding the infant, and locally available foods can quite easily be prepared as weaning foods without having to resort either to purchased manufactured foods or food handouts.

However, where poverty and malnutrition exist, and especially in urban or densely populated rural areas, supplementary feeding programmes may be useful in the control of childhood malnutrition. Unless supplementary foods and supplementary feeding programmes are either highly subsidized or provided free to poor families, they will fail to help the most vulnerable group of the population. Marketed protein-rich supplements, which are more expensive than local cereals, legumes or dried fish, have no benefit for the poor and may be a waste of money to those who buy them.

Supplementary feeding programmes are only palliatives, and do not correct the underlying causes of malnutrition. It must be carefully considered whether the high expense involved could not be better spent on programmes that would more effectively prevent malnutrition or attack its root causes.

Foods used in supplementary feeding programmes should be locally produced as far as possible; they should fit in with cultural food habits and practices, meet nutritional needs, and be considered in the context of the existing food and nutrition conditions of families in the area. Wherever possible supplementary feeding programmes should include nutrition education.

Nutrition education

This is an important strategy that needs to be given increased attention in most countries. The basis of any nutrition education programme should be to encourage the consumption of a nutritionally adequate diet and to stimulate effective demand for appropriate foods.

In the past, however, nutrition education has too often been conducted in a singularly unimaginative way. People have been instructed to eat this or that food because it is "good for you". As a result there are very few examples of successful nutrition education programmes. These "do good" programmes have frequently been carried out by persons of a different culture from those being educated. Attempts have often been made to make radical changes in the diets of the people who are the targets of the nutrition education.

It is stressed that nutrition educators should take as their first premise, to be included in their first "lesson", a recognition that most mothers are doing their best to feed their families properly.

An inadequate total intake of food by young children (an energy deficiency) is the main cause of malnutrition in Africa. Therefore, initial advice might be to continue feeding the infant with the same food as before but to do this more frequently or to provide just a little more of the food. This advice should be more acceptable to parents than the attempt to make major, often unrealistic changes in the diet.

The other changes in nutrition recommended should be simple and feasible for the family, be consistent with its cultural habits and of course be nutritionally sound.

Nutrition education has frequently failed because the advice did not conform with the above criteria. Throughout the world there are examples of nutrition education messages that urge poor mothers to provide their child with meat or fish every day, or one egg a day, or three cups of milk per day. This may make "dietary" or "nutritional" sense but in all other respects it is senseless. Except in a very few communities and countries, poor families cannot afford to feed these foods to their young children so often. There are cheap alternatives described elsewhere in this manual, the legumes being particularly good examples.

Nutrition education in a country is carried out by several ministries (health, agriculture, education, social or community development, etc.) and may also be performed by various nongovernmental organizations. All these bodies should agree on common objectives for a nutrition education programme, and each ministry must decide how it plans to implement it. Factors that should be decided upon, and that rarely are clearly defined, include the content of the message (discussed above), the audience that the programme is targeted to reach, and the media to be used. Again, this appears simple but in the author's experience it will require a change in both the philosophy and operation of most nutrition education programmes in Africa.

In general it may be wise to use a combination of communication media; a concentrated campaign using the radio may, however, be the cheapest and most effective way of reaching the large bulk of the population. In addition to stations controlled by the government, commercial radio (and television) should be used for nutrition education. Certain priority issues or areas of concern should receive concentrated effort. As mentioned, the stress should be on small changes that will complement existing dietary practices and not on major changes. In the past, failure has occurred because an attempt has been made to impart a mass of general information on nutrition, rather than hitting hard with a few well-designed messages in a limited number of priority areas.

The efforts of the various ministries and organizations should be closely coordinated so that the messages received by families from different sources will complement and reinforce each other — sometimes different agencies provide conflicting advice.

Answers to such questions as, Who should give nutrition education? When should it be offered? and, To whom should it be aimed? are in general quite simple. Everyone who has the knowledge (members of health teams, school teachers, agricultural extension workers) should provide nutrition education. They should do this at every possible opportunity (for example, the doctor when he is treating a patient, the midwife at the antenatal clinic, the health nurse as she visits a home, the extension officer at a farmers' meeting or *baraza*, the school teacher in a class or at a parents' meeting). Every person in the country should be the target of nutrition education. Even if the topic or the message concerns the problem of protein-energy malnutrition in the pre-school child, this is so important that all people can benefit from being informed about it. Priority points for nutrition education in many African countries might include:

- More frequent feeding of young children with existing foods;
- Increased amounts of foods at each meal for children during the weaning and post-weaning period;
- Greater consumption by children of whatever legumes are available and commonly consumed by the family;
- Inclusion of foods such as groundnuts that are rich in protein and provide a concentrated source of energy;
- Encouragement of breast-feeding and discouragement of bottle-feeding (i.e., the protection and promotion of breast-feeding);
- Increased use of foods rich in carotene (dark green leafy vegetables, yellow fruits and vegetables) by young children in areas where vitamin A deficiency is a problem;
- Attendance by pregnant women at clinics where iron and other supplements are available and where the progress of pregnancy can be checked;
- Encouragement of families to attend with their young children at under-fives and similar clinics, and to follow the growth of their children;
- Provision of information about the need for immunizations and where these can be obtained;
- Information that will help to reduce infectious diseases, which often contribute to malnutrition.

These examples are not all applicable to all communities or countries, but each is practical and appropriate for many areas of Africa.

Perhaps the most persistent and frequent error that has been made in nutrition education in Africa and elsewhere has been the overriding attention given to animal protein. It is now generally agreed that protein is not the main deficiency to be overcome, and that even if it were, animal products do not offer a reasonable or feasible solution in most of Africa. Protein-energy malnutrition, which is the most important nutritional problem, is much more often due to a low total intake of food by the child who may then be deficient both in energy and protein. The solution is to increase the quantity of foods already eaten. If efforts are to be made to increase protein intake then the stress should be on vegetable foods, such as legumes, that are rich in protein, rather than on animal products. Yet in so many nutrition education programmes of the last 20 years vast and wasted emphasis has been placed on increasing the consumption of meat, fish, milk, eggs and manufactured protein-rich foods. This education has totally failed because the objective was wrong, economic reasons precluded the adoption of the advice and frequently the foods recommended were not easily available.

Nutrition educators have much to learn from commercial advertising, which has often been successful in changing food habits and attitudes. Unfortunately the advertisers have often caused changes that have had bad nutritional consequences. The commercial firms have shown that their methods can get poor people to purchase nutritionally useless products like sodas and colas, and to switch from breast-feeding to bottle-feeding with often disastrous consequences for the infant. This commercial promotion skilfully uses the media. The commercial talent available should more often be harnessed to assist with nutrition and health education.

33. EVALUATION OF NUTRITION PROGRAMMES [1]

Public-health and nutrition programmes are frequently conducted without any plans for their evaluation. A campaign to increase the number of toilets constructed, a policy to triple the number of under-fives clinics, a new school-feeding programme and increased emphasis on nutrition education may all be important activities in a country, but are seldom adequately evaluated.

---

[1] This chapter is largely based on a book by Latham (FAO, 1972), which also provides more information both on planning and evaluation of the coordinated integrated nutrition activities that came to be known as "applied nutrition programmes", or ANPS.

Evaluation simply consists of appraising, measuring or judging the progress made by a programme or activity toward its stated objectives. The government that supports a programme, the workers who implement it and the people who are the beneficiaries should all be interested to know how effective any programme is.

An integral part of all applied nutrition activities should be some form of evaluation.

Because evaluation includes a determination of progress toward certain objectives there are two basic prerequisites for useful evaluation. First is the need to have stated, preferably in writing, the objectives of the programmes. Second is the need for some base-line data, however simple.

In other words there is a need to know the position before the programme begins and to have some statement of what changes are expected to occur as a result of the programme.

This may sound theoretical or complex but in fact it can be quite simple. For example, a supplementary feeding programme may be established at a health unit with the purpose of rehabilitating moderate cases of malnutrition who have marked growth retardation. The objective, broadly stated, might be to improve the nutritional status of 30-50 children attending the unit over a 3-month period. But in order to allow for a meaningful evaluation it is preferable to state the objectives more specifically and in an easily measurable form. One specific objective might be to improve the percentage weight-for-age by 10 percent over a 3-month period of at least 80 percent of children whose initial weight-for-age was less than 70 percent of the expected. The base-line data consist here of the weight-for-age of each child when first seen at the unit. The follow-up information needed for the evaluation is the weight of children 3 months later.

Other simple examples of evaluation are the assessment of the nutrition knowledge of mothers before and after receiving health education, the weight gains of infants before and after attending under-fives clinics, the protein intake of families before and after a campaign to increase legume production and consumption, and the percentage of mothers breast-feeding their babies at 6 months of age before and after a campaign in an urban area where the majority of women have begun to bottle-feed their infants.

Uses

Evaluation is useful in several different ways. First, it helps the worker to know how he is getting on with the job and it may suggest ways of improving his work or accelerating progress. It may suggest that certain actions produce good results and others do not. This may lead the worker to concentrate on the useful activities and modify, reorient or even abandon the unproductive ones, thus speeding advancement toward the objectives set.

Secondly, evaluation is useful for the other members of the team and for the programme planners. They can analyse the evaluation reports from all the different workers in the programme and obtain a measure of overall progress and of the relative contribution of each component or activity. This facilitates logical planning and may lead to some revision of the programme operation.

Thirdly, evaluation provides the general public — the people whom the scheme is designed to help — with an indication of what has been achieved. Because community support is essential to the success of a programme, it is incumbent on the workers to let those receiving help know how the programme is progressing. This is similar to a company or business, which must from time to time let its shareholders know how the business is doing. Unless people are shown and made to understand what is happening to them, and the role they themselves are playing in the change, much of the value of a programme may be lost. By understanding the results achieved, the public might well be encouraged to cooperate more fully and to assist in programme activities. Evaluation might also convince them and their leaders that some aspect of the programme about which they were sceptical is producing results. For example, in an area where there was little enthusiasm about school feeding, parents might be greatly influenced to support it financially and with self-help activities if they were provided with clearly understandable evidence showing that children getting meals grew better, learned more and were less prone to absenteeism.

Evaluation is therefore a constructive process that can gain more support for the programme from the government, from outside agencies and from the public. It can also encourage the worker and help him to be more effective and efficient.

Time-scale

In some activities evaluation consists of a measurement before and after completion of action. The difference between the two measurements indicates the change occurring during the period of the action; it may or may not be entirely produced by the action.

This type of cut-and-dried measure is not suitable for most applied nutrition programmes, although the technique may be used for their individual components.

216

In any broadly based applied nutrition programme it is very important that evaluation should be taking place continuously throughout the whole period of operation.

Evaluation of all the project activities serves to show up the weak links in the overall programme and, if continuously done, remedial action can be taken at an early stage, either by correcting some fault or by reorienting the programme.

Personnel

Although there are exceptions, the major part of evaluation should generally be carried out by those working on the spot and not by visiting experts.

The advantage of this far outweighs the disadvantages. Admittedly the project worker is a biased person; he is measuring the effects of his own work and is therefore likely to exaggerate his successes and minimize his failures. Because of his familiarity and involvement with his work, he cannot look objectively and critically at the activities of the programme. In contrast, an outsider coming specially to evaluate has no axe to grind, for it is not to his advantage or disadvantage to report progress or lack of it. He is therefore more impartial and fairer than the local worker. The expert from outside may also have more technical competence and even more time to evaluate the programme than the local worker.

However, the disadvantages of evaluation by an outsider are many. In the first place he has not the same knowledge of conditions and of the people as has the local worker. Where change in people is taking place, this is of great importance. The local worker is known and if he has done his job properly he is trusted as a friend and a helper. The danger of an outsider coming in is that he may create the impression that his purpose is to study the local people or that he is conducting some experiment on them for his own purposes. This is particularly so if medical examinations include taking samples of blood, urine and stools. Many people are suspicious of outsiders and are unwilling to cooperate until they feel they can trust then and clearly understand their motives.

A second major difficulty for the outsider is that the workers and the public (who are often loyal to the project) may consider evaluation by an outsider as checking up on the programme, and therefore as a search for shortcomings.

In some circumstances outside help is needed in evaluation. This must be carefully used, with attempts made to minimize the disadvantages mentioned previously. The outsider may, for example, be extremely useful in advising on the type of data that could be collected and might assist with its analysis. The actual collection of the data would then be left to the local worker.

In some applied nutrition programmes it might be decided that certain necessary measurements are technically beyond the capability of the project workers to obtain. Occasionally also the measurements to be made require special apparatus or instruments that are not available to the programme staff.

Where field workers are not trained in statistics, at certain stages in the programme outside assistance on statistical work may prove invaluable. The provision of one or more trained persons to help with the tabulation of data and its statistical analysis may take a great load of work off their shoulders. It may also result in a more valid and accurate analysis of data collected. This type of outside help is unobtrusive and extremely useful.

34. PRACTICAL SOLUTIONS TO NUTRITION PROBLEMS

This summary of suggestions for practical solutions to nutritional problems is by no means complete. It merely attempts to list ideas concerning the improvement of nutrition that are suitable for adaptation by a nation, a village, or by individuals in a community. Each area and each community has its own problems that must be tackled at local level. The suggestions made here can therefore not be expected to do more than stimulate thought.

It is clear that many of the solutions are educational, for again and again it has been stressed that one of the main causes of poor nutrition in Africa is a lack of knowledge about food. Many other suggestions are basically agricultural in nature. This manual is not designed to give details either on teaching methods or of agricultural practice. Information on increasing and improving food production must be sought in manuals of agriculture, horticulture, animal husbandry, fisheries and poultry keeping.

Improving nutritional knowledge

Lack of knowledge is an important cause of malnutrition in Africa. Nutrition knowledge can for example be improved by:

a. Education — nutrition education in schools, in literacy classes, in farmer-training centres, and in village meetings (see Fig. 59).

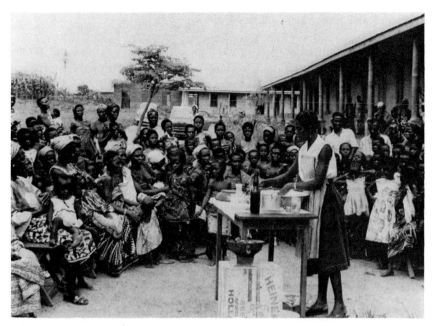

FIGURE 59. Cooking demonstration in a village.

b. Personal example — government ministers and respected leaders might include the topic of nutrition in their speeches and might consume controversial but nutritionally desirable food in public.

c. Distribution of pamphlets and posters featuring material on nutrition in newspapers, publicizing nutrition facts through radio broadcasts, and at agricultural and other shows.

d. Demonstrations — actual demonstrations of the preparation and cooking of food, especially food suitable for children. This can be done by health nurses in health centres and clinics, by community development workers and by domestic-science teachers in schools.

e. Team approach — coordination of effort to disseminate nutrition knowledge through district and village committees.

f. Encouraging nutritionally good traditional food habits, e.g., the eating of lake flies, *mchicha*, and wild fruits.

g. Discouraging undesirable food habits, e.g., taboos against eggs and fish.

h. Teaching mothers good practical weaning habits, e.g., use of sour milk in gruel, pounded groundnuts for infants, and vegetable mixtures.

i. Banning by legislation the advertising of milk for bottle-feeding.

219

Increasing and improving food production

Increasing and improving food production is mainly an agricultural problem. Aims should be:

a. To promote an overall increase to ensure a sufficient energy supply, with emphasis on having enough available for times of intense agricultural activity at the end of the season, i.e., during the usual "hungry period".
b. To increase production of plants that are good sources of protein. Every household should grow more beans, groundnuts, cowpeas, etc.
c. To increase and improve production of animal protein by:
— Better animal husbandry;
— More use of cattle and goats as a source of food rather than of prestige;
— Use of goat's milk;
— Improved and increased poultry keeping and use of eggs, especially as a food for toddlers and young children;
— Increased and improved methods of catching and preserving fish;
— The construction of village and household fishponds (see Fig. 54) in all areas where perennial water exists[1];
— The wider use of dams as a source of fish production;
— Extensive use of small animals, especially pigeons, guinea pigs and rabbits for food;
— Greater use of sea urchins, locusts, lake flies, etc., as food;
— Wider use of meat from game animals, including controlled cropping and game farming.
d. To increase vegetable and fruit production, especially to ensure adequate intake of vitamins A and C by:
— A policy of encouraging backyard gardens (or a vegetable garden near every home);
— Allocation of land allotments for growing food in towns;
— Establishment of school, village, and community orchards and gardens.

Improving food distribution

Food should be equitably distributed. This does not necessarily happen even in those places where sufficient food is available. More equitable distribution can be achieved by:

---

[1] Improperly maintained fishponds can lead to an increase in malaria and schistosomiasis (bilharzia). Public-health advice should be sought and steps taken to prevent mosquitoes and snails from breeding.

a. Improving communications to ensure that excess stocks in one area reach another area short of that commodity.

b. Better trading facilities, i.e., by more food markets and shops; better stocks of nutritionally valuable manufactured and preserved foods in village shops at reasonable prices; improved market places; and more cooperative-type food shops.

c. Fair distribution within the family to ensure a fair share of protein-rich and other foods for children, and increased supplies of food for pregnant and lactating women.

d. Instituting midday meals for day-school children; encouraging children to take food to school; supplying milk at school; improving meals in boarding schools.

e. Making available special foods for young children; developing special recipes for toddlers.

f. Paying wages weekly instead of monthly; encouraging better family budgeting.

g. Ensuring availability of midday meals for workers, subsidized canteens, rations for labourers.

Improving food and crop storage

An estimated 25 percent of all food produced in Africa may never be consumed by man. Instead it spoils or is eaten by insects, rats and other pests. Measures to correct this situation can be taken in the fields, in the household, and in the shops and warehouses. These may include:

a. Control of rats by trapping, poison, rat-proofing grain stores, etc.

b. Control of insects by use of insecticides, better food stores (see Fig. 60), airtight food containers.

c. Control of fungus and food rot by storage of food in as dry a state as possible, and by use of better containers.

d. Control of birds by destruction, especially in millet and wheat areas.

e. Protective measures against monkeys, baboons, porcupines, wild pigs, and other destructive animals, even elephants.

Improving food processing

Proper food processing can ensure that nutrient values of food are maintained at the highest possible level and that food surpluses are utilized. Suitable measures are:

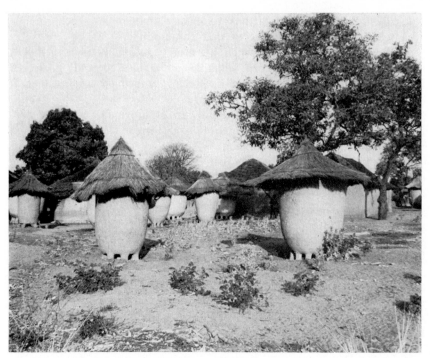

FIGURE 60   Efficient village granaries in the Ivory Coast.

a. Better methods of food preservation in the home and the village, e.g., drying or smoking of meat and fish, preservation of fruits and vegetables, home or village production of cheese.

b. Better cooking, e.g., less prolonged boiling of vegetables containing vitamin C, adding the minimal quantity of water to rice, preparing special dishes for infants.

c. Increased use of processes for preservation of local foods and in some instances for making them more palatable. This requires more small-scale commercial enterprise, e.g., commercial fish-drying, drying or canning of food products, and production plants to make an edible product from local soybeans.

d. Supply of well-processed milk products at reasonable cost.

e. Enrichment of highly milled cereals with vitamins and iron. This can best be achieved by legislation.

f. Iodization of salt to prevent goitre.

g. Fluoridation of community waters to reduce dental caries in areas where this is feasible and where the water contains less than 0.5 parts per million of fluoride.

222

Practical steps for the health worker

In order to improve the nutritional status of local communities, the health worker should:

a. Provide a good curative service to treat persons suffering both from malnutrition and from the many diseases closely linked with malnutrition.

b. Take the opportunity with in- and outpatients of discussing and teaching the importance of a balanced diet. Stress especially the needs of children, and pregnant and lactating women.

c. Organize the efficient distribution of supplementary foods, where these are available for young children.

d. Encourage the use and proper keeping of "road-to-health" or weight charts of young children at clinics or even by household units.

e. Give food demonstrations at maternal and child-health clinics and elsewhere. Concentrate especially on suitable weaning-food mixtures for young children. Always try to use foodstuffs that are locally acceptable and available. Participation by the mothers in such demonstrations is important. Mothers can help prepare the food, can feed it to their infants during the demonstrations and in some cases can bring their own local foods. Examples of suitable demonstration foods are given in Section VI.

f. Take preventive measures against gastrointestinal disease, infections and other diseases that are precursors of malnutrition. This should include immunization against certain diseases.

g. Conduct investigations and surveys to ascertain the types of malnutrition occurring and their extent. The results of these will allow the health worker to give sound advice on remedial measures. Study local feeding practices and customs relating to food.

h. Take an active part in team activities designed to improve nutrition. If no committee or team exists in a village or area, the health worker might bring together his agricultural, education, and social development colleagues to form a representative team to tackle nutritional problems in a coordinated way.

i. Keep notes and record clinical details relating to nutrition.

j. Give advice regarding the existing diets of all the institutions in the area. Work out (using the tables in Appendix 3) the nutritive value of the diet. Then using Table 1 in Appendix 1, see if the diet falls short of requirements. If so, suggest improvements, using as far as possible local foods, without unduly raising the cost of the diet.

k. After studying the problem in each area and assessing its aetiology, take steps, using all available health personnel, voluntary workers and other staff, to improve infant and toddler feeding.

l. Encourage prolonged breast-feeding.

m. Discourage bottle-feeding of infants.

n. Encourage supplementation of breast milk with other foods, beginning from the fourth month.

o. Organize proper antenatal and postnatal clinics for women. Assess the incidence of anaemia and decide whether to give prophylactic iron preparations to all pregnant women.

p. Try to improve food hygiene in market, shop and home.

q. Take steps to improve food preparation in the home so as to minimize loss of nutrients.

VI. DIETS, TODDLER RECIPES AND HOME PRESERVATION OF FOOD

In each of the diets given in this section, specific foods are mentioned. They can be substituted, in many instances, by other similar foods of equivalent nutritive value. This may be desirable or necessary if the alternative food is cheaper, more easily available or better liked. Different amounts will be needed to produce the same effect, however.

Thus, for energy, the following amounts of mainly carbohydrate foods (uncooked) each supply approximately 1 000 Calories:

Food	*Amount (grams)*
Rice	325
Maize meal	325
Millet	350
Wheat flour	350
Dried cassava	350
Bread	500
Plantain	800
Yam	1 000
Sweet potato	1 000
Potato	1 350

Similarly, the following quantities of (uncooked) foods each provide approximately 10 g protein:

Food	*Amount (grams)*
Dried fish	16
Dried skim milk	27
Soybeans	28
Winged beans	30

Dried groundnuts	32
Fish (sea or freshwater)	40
Meat (beef, mutton, goat, poultry)	40
Kidney beans	42
Cowpeas	45
Chick-peas or pigeon peas	50
Eggs	75
Cereals (rice, wheat, maize)	100
Potatoes	500
Plantain	1 000
Cassava roots	1 200

Equivalent quantities for the different nutrients in various foods can be calculated using the food composition table in Appendix 3.

35. FEEDING THE FAMILY

Most of the food that people consume is eaten at home. Therefore faults in family feeding are the main causes of malnutrition in Africa. Exceptions include malnutrition in estate and other workers, and students who live away from home in workers' quarters, hostels and other institutions.

It was stated previously that apart from exceptional years and at the end of the agricultural season, people in tropical Africa on the whole have enough to eat; that is, enough to fill their stomachs and assuage hunger, and usually enough to satisfy their energy requirements. However, this sufficiency of food is usually composed of predominantly carbohydrate foods. In young children and in pregnant and lactating women, energy requirements are relatively high, so a large quantity of the staple carbohydrate food has to be eaten to satisfy these needs. If the food eaten is a cereal such as maize, rice, millet or wheat, and is lightly milled, then it will usually provide both sufficient energy and sufficient iron and B vitamins, though, in the case of maize, not enough to prevent pellagra. Foods other than the staple must provide the extra protein, fat, calcium, vitamin A and vitamin C required. Africans usually obtain adequate vitamin D from the action of sunlight on the skin.

The extra protein required may come from protein-rich vegetable foods such as beans, groundnuts, cowpeas, soybeans, lentils, or other legumes. Some may come from animal products such as meat, fish, milk, and eggs.

226

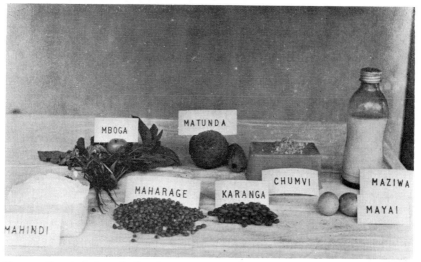

FIGURE 61. A balanced diet for one person for one day contains foods from each column on page 228, (I) maize *(mahindi)* is a carbohydrate-rich food, (II) (A) beans *(maharage)* and groundnuts *(karanga)* have vegetable protein, (B) milk *(maziwa)* and eggs *(mayai)* have animal protein, (III) fruit *(matunde)* and vegetables *(mboga)* contain vitamin C and carotene. Fat occurs in the groundnuts, which, together with beans and maize, provide B vitamins. Salt *(chumvi)* is also desirable.

If the main foodstuff in the diet is bananas, cassava, sweet potatoes or some other starchy food, then an even greater quantity of additional protein is necessary than in the case of a diet based on a cereal grain.

A mixture of vegetable foods, such as two cereals and a legume (e.g., maize, millet, and cowpeas) or a root, a cereal and a legume (e.g., cassava, sorghum, and groundnuts) eaten at one meal provide better-quality protein together than larger quantities of a single vegetable food would. This is because the mixture usually contains all the essential amino acids whereas a single cereal, root or legume is usually deficient in one or more of the essential amino acids.

A family eating good quantities of legumes and occasional animal protein foods in addition to their cereal, banana or root staple probably satisfy their requirements for energy, iron, protein and B vitamins. Fat is also added to the diet if the legumes include good quantities of groundnuts or soybeans, or if the animal protein consists of fatty meat, fish, milk or eggs.

The above diet is lacking only in vitamin A and vitamin C. These can best be supplied by fresh fruit and vegetables. Many of these items contain vitamin C and carotene, the precursor of vitamin A. The dark green leaves also provide much iron and some calcium.

227

Every family should be advised to put the above principles into practice so that all its members have a satisfactory diet. This can be achieved if they consume daily, or, better still, at every meal, a reasonable quantity of food from each column in the lists given below. This assures the variety so important for a balanced diet (see Fig. 61):

I	II	III
Carbohydrate-rich foods	Protein-rich foods	Foods containing Vitamin C and/or carotene
Cereals:	Vegetable origin:	Fresh vegetables, including green leaves
maize	beans	
millet	peas	Fresh fruit, including wild fruit
rice	groundnuts	
teff	soybeans	
wheat	lentils	
	cowpeas, etc.	
Starchy foods:	Animal origin:	
bananas		
cassava	meat	
potatoes	eggs	
yams	fish	
	milk and milk products	
	insects, etc.	

A certain amount of fat is desirable. This may be bought as cooking fat, or may be obtained in the diet from milk, groundnuts, etc. If the main staple of the diet is a highly refined cereal, as opposed to a home-pounded or lightly milled one, then extra vitamin B-containing foods should be consumed.

Seven examples of family diets based on the above information are given below. In each instance the amount given is that which should be eaten by an average man. The amounts can be varied for women and children by using Table 1 in Appendix 1 and the food composition table in Appendix 3. Extras such as sugar, spices, tea and other beverages are not included since, although they make the diet more palatable, they add little of nutritive value. The localities mentioned refer to places in East Africa where this type of diet might be eaten. They are not average diets in these areas, but are suggestions as to what would constitute a satisfactory diet.

228

Area	Food	Amount (grams/head/day)
1. Kenya coast	Rice	500
	Fish	100
	Beans	150
	Amaranth (*mchicha*)	100
	Mango	100
	Coconut	50
	Oil	15
	Salt	15
2. Buganda village	Plantains (cooking bananas)	1 000
	Sweet potatoes	200
	Meat	50
	Beans	150
	Sweet potato leaves	150
	Tomatoes	50
	Oil	15
	Salt	10
3. Morogoro Region, Tanzania	Maize (*dona*)	500
	Dried sprats (*dagaa*)	50
	Cowpeas	100
	Amaranth (*mchicha*)	100
	Oranges	100
	Onions	50
	Oil	15
	Salt	10
4. Nairobi, Kenya	White wheat-bread	400
	Rice	100
	Eggs	30
	Meat	100
	Carrots	100
	Green leaves	50
	Butter or margarine	25
	Fresh bananas	100
	Milk (in tea)	60
	Sugar	30
	Salt	10
5. Central Region, Tanzania	Millet	400
	Cassava	200
	Sour milk	150
	Tomatoes	100
	Sesame leaves	100
	Groundnuts	50
	Bambara nuts	75
	Baobab fruit	30
	Salt	10

229

Area	Food	Amount (grams/head/day)
6. Lake Victoria shore	Maize (*sembe*)	600
	Fish	100
	Cowpeas	150
	Papaya	150
	Vegetables (mixed)	200
	Groundnuts	75
	Oil	20
	Salt	10
7. Masailand	Milk	2 000
	Blood (animal)	100
	Maize	150
	Wild leaves	100
	Wild fruit	100
	Bananas	200
	Salt	15

Vegetable mixtures

Where foods of animal origin are not often available the quality of the protein in the diet can be improved by providing a mixture or variety of vegetable products at each meal. Thus if a household has maize and beans available it is far better nutritionally to eat some of both at each meal rather than to eat maize for two weeks and then beans for two weeks. The former is frequently practised by many people in East Africa. For example, *irio*, a traditional Kikuyu food, includes maize, beans, potato, and green leaves, and the Kamba food *isyo* is a mixture of whole-kernel maize with beans and sometimes vegetables. Examples of vegetable mixtures are given below, some of which are traditional dishes. The various foods do not have to be physically mixed together, but can just as well be eaten separately at the same meal.

— Rice and bean stew.
— Beans and boiled maize (*nyoyo*).
— Maize, beans and green leafy vegetables.
— Baked sweet potatoes served with peas or beans and amaranth leaves.
— *Uji* or *ugali* made from one part cassava flour, two parts maize flour, and served with sauce made from cowpeas and tomatoes.
— Sorghum gruel and bananas with groundnut paste.
— Millet served with onion, yam, peas and tomato relish.
— Groundnut soup (see recipe No. 12, p. 234) with potatoes.

230

— Sesame (simsim), groundnuts served with *ugali*.
— Vegetable stew (green leaves, tomatoes, peas and onion) served with rice or *ugali*.
— Cassava with bean mush (see recipe No. 13, p. 234).
— Plantains with beans and cabbage.

36. RECIPES FOR INFANTS AND YOUNG CHILDREN

The role of various nutrients in the diets of infants and young children has been described elsewhere in this book. The importance of introducing new foods to supplement breast and other milk from the fifth or sixth month of life has been stressed. Here, 18 examples of special dishes suitable for infants and young children are given. There are of course innumerable other recipes, and for each family the foods used will depend on local custom and what is available.

Dishes suitable for weaning, and for toddlers and young children

1. GRUEL (*uji*) WITH BEANS OR GROUNDNUTS

Ingredients: Flour made from maize, millet, cassava, or rice.
                  Bean mush (see recipe 13) or groundnut soup (see recipe 12).
Method: Prepare a gruel in the customary way. While it is simmering in the pot, add bean mush or thick groundnut soup. Stir vigorously. Cook for 2 to 5 minutes. Remove the gruel from the fire or stove. Cool and serve to infant or young child.

2. GRUEL WITH SOUR (OR FRESH) MILK

Ingredients: Flour from maize, millet, cassava, rice, etc.
                  $\frac{1}{2}$ cup sour (or fresh) milk.
Method: Prepare a gruel in the customary way. While it is simmering in the pot, add $\frac{1}{2}$ of sour (or fresh) milk. Stir and serve when sufficiently cool.

3. GRUEL WITH DRIED SKIM MILK POWDER

Ingredients: Flour made from maize, millet, cassava, rice, etc.
Dried skim milk (DSM) powder.

Method: Add one tablespoonful of milk powder to each cup of flour and mix. Add sugar or salt as required. Prepare a gruel in the normal way for feeding the infant or child.

4. SCRAMBLED EGG

Ingredients: 1 egg.
1 tablespoonful of milk (optional).
Pinch of salt.
$\frac{1}{2}$ teaspoonful oil or fat.

Method: Break egg into cup and beat with spoon or fork. Add milk and salt and stir again. Put pan or pot on fire and add oil. When hot, add egg mixture from cup. Stir gently until it is a semi-solid creamy consistency. Serve alone or mixed with *uji* to child.

5. BOILED EGG

Ingredients: 1 egg.

Method: Put egg (in shell) into pot containing enough cold water to cover it. Put on fire and remove egg when water boils. Remove shell and mash egg in cup or plate. Serve alone or mixed with *uji* to infant.

6. EGG IN A SIEVE

Ingredients: 1 egg.

Method: Break egg into sieve. Put sieve into or just above pot of boiling water. Cook until egg begins to set. Serve to child.

7. PAPAYA MUSH

Ingredients: 1 papaya.
Fresh milk or DSM (optional).

Method: Take a slice of ripe papaya. Remove pips and skin. Mash it in bowl or on plate. Add and mix 4 tablespoonfuls of milk or 1 tablespoonful DSM powder, if available. Serve to infant or child.

8. BANANA MUSH

Ingredients: 2 ripe bananas.
½ cupful fresh or sour milk or 1 tablespoonful DSM.

Method: Peel bananas and mash with fork or rub through sieve. Add milk or milk powder. Stir and mix. Spoon-feed to infant or child. (This dish can also be made using cooked green bananas or plantains.)

9. AMARANTH (*mchicha*) WITH EGG

Ingredients: Handful of amaranth or other edible leaves.
1 egg.
1 teaspoonful of oil (optional).

Method: Wash amaranth leaves and remove stalks. Put in pot of boiling water together with egg in its shell. Remove both when leaves are tender (after 5 minutes). Cut up leaves finely. Remove shell from egg and mash egg. Mix egg and leaf mush together adding ½ teaspoonful oil, if available. Serve alone or mixed with gruel to infant.

10. VEGETABLE MUSH

Ingredients: Handful edible leaves.
1 carrot (optional).
1 tomato (optional).

Method: Take some cooked green leaves and one cooked carrot, if available, from family pot. Rub through sieve. Take ripe tomato, if available, and rub through sieve. Mix and feed to infant or mix with cooked mashed potato or *uji* before feeding.

11. LIVER PASTE

Ingredients: 50 grams liver.
Pinch of salt.

Method: Cook liver in usual way. Cut into small pieces. Force as much as possible through sieve. Add salt. Feed to infant or child. (Other meat can be cooked for the child in the same way.)

12. GROUNDNUT SOUP

Ingredients: $\frac{1}{2}$ cup groundnuts.
Pinch of salt.

Method: Roast groundnuts until pale brown. Remove skins. Crush groundnuts with pestle and mortar (or on a stone). Add salt. Mix with water to form paste. Cook for 10 minutes in small quantity of water. Serve alone or mixed with gruel to child.

13. BEAN (OR OTHER LEGUME) MUSH

Ingredients: 50 grams beans or other legumes.

Method: Soak beans overnight. Boil in usual way. Mash with fork or spoon. Force through sieve, removing skins. Feed with maize or other gruel to child.

14. FISH PORRIDGE

Ingredients: 50 grams dried fish.
Gruel of staple food.

Method: Take 5-10 dried sprats (*dagaa*). Crush and pound without removing bones. Add to simmering gruel and cook for 10 minutes. Serve to child. If larger dried fish is used, head, tail and bones should be removed.

15. GROUNDNUT AND BANANA MUSH

Ingredients: 1 banana.
1 handful groundnuts.

Method: Roast groundnuts and remove skin. Boil or roast banana. Put groundnuts and banana in mortar and pound. When mush is a fine, smooth consistency, feed to child.

16. AVOCADO MUSH

Ingredients: $\frac{1}{2}$ avocado pear (ripe).
$\frac{1}{2}$ orange (optional).

Method: Remove skin and stone from the avocado. Mash up flesh with spoon or fork. Add juice from $\frac{1}{2}$ orange (if available) and mix. Serve to infant.

234

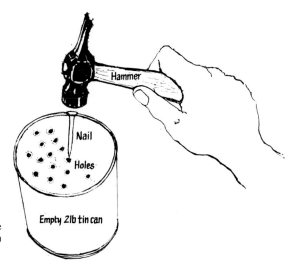

FIGURE 62. A simple sieve can be made from an empty tin can.

17. RICE AND BEAN GRUEL

Ingredients: 50 grams beans (or other legume).
               120 grams rice.
Method: Boil beans or take a portion from beans cooked for adults. Remove skins and crush through sieve. Take cooked rice from adult meal. Mash with wooden spoon until soft and creamy. Add beans and mix. Serve to infant or child.

18. MILLET WITH BEANS OR COWPEAS

Ingredients: 120 grams millet (or other cereal) flour.
               50 grams beans or cowpeas.
               Pinch of salt.
Method: Cook finely ground millet flour into gruel or thin porridge. Soak beans overnight and simmer in water with salt. Crush through sieve. Mix with millet gruel and serve to infant.

As can be seen from the above recipes, a wire sieve is useful in preparing infant foods. It serves to change a solid lumpy food into one of fine, soft consistency, suitable for a child with few or no teeth. If a sieve is not available, one can easily be made by punching 20-30 holes in the bottom of an empty tin with a medium-sized nail. This makes a perfectly adequate sieve (see Fig. 62), but it should be carefully washed after use.

235

Many adult dishes, after being put through a sieve, are suitable and good for young children. It must be remembered, however, that spices, especially those that have a burning hot taste, are unsuitable. Dishes containing curry powder, hot peppers, etc. should be avoided.

In this book no attempt has been made to produce a weaning chart or daily menus for children of different ages. Tables of this kind tend to be too dogmatic and may prevent both teachers and mothers from thinking out for themselves what is the desirable food in each instance. It is better that each family, and each infant, be treated individually, receiving a diet based or sound nutritional principles. Advice on diets should always be realistic and adapted to the foods most commonly used and most easily available.

As has been stated, breast-feeding should, under most circumstances, continue for as long as possible. With an infant who has developed satisfactorily, supplementary feeding should begin between the fourth and sixth month. In some circumstances, it is desirable to begin mixed feeding earlier than the fifth month. A gruel of the local staple with added milk is an excellent food on which to start mixed feeding. If milk is not available then any legume can be used instead. It should at first be given in one feeding a day, using a spoon and cup. After a week or two, when the child has become accustomed to semi-solid food, other dishes can be introduced. Next might come mashed fruit (e.g., mashed papaya) or vegetables, or possibly tomato or orange juice. A week or two later, some different foods can be tried while continuing the others. These may be groundnut soup, or bean mush or a fish dish (see recipes 12, 13, 14). At this stage, semi-solid food might form part of two feedings a day.

By the end of the first year, all or any of the types of food in the recipes could have been tried, breast-feeding all the while. The infant should also by this time have been given the experience of trying many of the adult dishes of the family, avoiding only obviously unsuitable foods, such as hot (peppery) curries, and alcoholic beverages.

During the period from 12 to 24 months, the infant can cope with many family dishes, but should receive more frequent meals than adults, and have proportionately larger quantities of proteins and some other nutrients (see Table 1 in Appendix 1). A number of the suggested recipes can continue to supplement the family food and breast milk that the toddler receives.

After the second year, breast-feeding will usually have ceased, and extra protein-rich foods will be especially important. The child will now be able to cope with most of the family food, but must get more than would appear to be his fair share. Extra dishes such as some of the suggested recipes are highly desirable during this pre-school period. The

236

young child may need more frequent feeding (four or more meals a day) than the adult members of the family.

Nursery schools, day-care centres and kindergartens

In Africa there is an increasing number of nursery schools, day-care centres and kindergartens where children from 1 to 6 years of age can be left while their mothers work, or which are established as pre-primary schools. Children attending such institutions should receive a daily meal consisting of food rich in those nutrients likely to be deficient in the home diet. The toddlers could with advantage be supplied with a protein-rich dish taken from one of the 18 recipes given in this chapter. Milk, if available, is a useful addition.

Older children should be given a properly balanced midday meal similar to those suggested in the next chapter for primary school children. Every effort should be made to provide nutrition education for the mothers who bring their children to these institutions. Mothers could be asked to help with meal preparations and would thus get first-hand experience of preparing nutritious dishes for young children.

37. INSTITUTIONAL DIETS

School

Primary day school. The importance of a midday meal at day schools and of a good balanced diet at boarding schools has been discussed in Chapter 8. Some suggestions for a suitable midday meal at a primary day school are given below.

Food	Amount (grams/head/meal)
1. Maize (*dona*) or rice	200
Meat or dried fish (*dagaa*)	30
Mixed vegetables	50
Green leaves	25
Beans or groundnuts	50
Sugar	10
Milk (full-cream powder)	10
Oil (red palm)	10
Salt	5

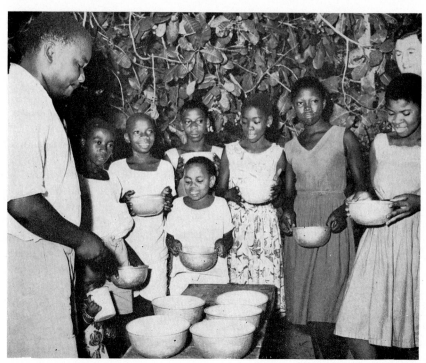

FIGURE 63. School feeding. A cold lunch may be as nutritious as a hot lunch.

Food	Amount (grams/head/meal)
2. Bananas (plantains)	400
Groundnuts	50
Mixed vegetables	50
Beans	50
Milk powder (DSM)	20
Oil (red palm)	10
Salt	5
3. Cassava flour	150
Millet	100
Meat or fish	50
Beans	100
Green leaves	75
Fruit	100
Oil (red palm)	10
Salt	5

Food	Amount (grams/head/meal)
4. Bread	150
Potatoes	150
Tomato	75
Onions	50
Beans	100
Fruit	75
Oil (red palm)	10
Salt	5

For a secondary day school the same foodstuffs could be provided, but the amount of each item should be increased by about 25 percent.

Occasionally one hears that for a school lunch to be nutritious it must include a hot dish. This is not true. Heat has nothing to do with nutritive quality. A cold lunch may be as nutritious as a hot lunch. It is the food served that determines the nutritive value of the meal (see Fig. 63).

Secondary boarding schools. The quantities of food given below are suitable per pupil per day. They should be divided up and served as three meals. Items such as meat, for which small daily amounts are indicated, may be given, say, twice a week in larger amounts (for example, 20 grams of meat per day make 140 grams per week, which can be given in two equal portions of 70 grams on Sunday and Wednesday).

Food	Amount (grams/head/day)
1. Maize (dona)	500
Rice	100
Beans	150
Groundnuts	100
Meat	20
Sprats, dried (dagaa)	20
Leafy vegetables	150
Sugar	30
Milk powder (DSM)	20
Oil (red palm)	20
Salt	10

Food	Amount (grams/head/day)
2. Bananas (plantains)	600
Potatoes	400
Rice	150
Meat	20
Beans	150
Groundnuts	50
Mixed vegetables	150
Fruit	100
Sugar	50
Milk (full-cream powder)	50
Oil (red palm)	10
Salt	10
3. Cassava flour	300
Millet	150
Green leaves	150
Fruit	100
Cowpeas	150
Groundnuts	100
Fish	50
Milk powder (DSM)	50
Oil (red palm)	10
Salt	10
4. Rice	300
Potatoes	150
Maize	100
Bread	150
Meat	50
Egg	30
Vegetables (mixed)	150
Margarine	50
Sugar	50
Fruit	150
Lentils	75
Groundnuts	50
Jam	30
Oil (red palm)	20
Milk (fresh)	0.5 litre
Salt	10

In a primary boarding school, the same foods could be provided but with an all-round reduction of about 25 percent in quantity.

240

Hospital feeding

Hospital patients usually spend most of their time in bed. Their need for energy is therefore reduced compared with active persons of the same sex, age and weight. However, they may have increased nutritional requirements because they enter hospital undernourished; they are pregnant, lactating or have recently had a baby; or their disease requires a special diet or extra nutrients. A suitable diet would be as follows:

Food	Amount (grams/head/day)
Bread	100
Maize (*dona*)	200
Rice	150
Meat	100
Vegetables	150
Fruit	150
Legumes	100
Milk (full-cream powder)	75 (or 0.5 litre fresh milk)
Oil (red palm)	20
Salt	10

Prison

A prison should provide a completely balanced diet suitable for persons doing heavy work. The diet should be cheap and simple. In some countries the scale of prison rations is laid down by law. In Tanzania each prisoner receives one 50-mg tablet of niacin per week in addition to the diet laid down. This measure was instituted to prevent the occurrence of pellagra. A suitable prison diet would be as follows:

Food	Amount (grams/head/day)
Maize (*dona*)	750
Beans	150
Green vegetables	150
Groundnuts	100
Meat	20
Sweet potatoes	50
Fruit	100
Salt	10
Oil (red palm)	5

The maize could be substituted by an equivalent amount of rice or millet.

Army

Food	Amount (grams/head/day)
Maize (*sembe* or *dona*)	400
Rice (unpolished)	100
Bread	100
Potatoes	400
Beans	100
Vegetables (mixed)	150
Onions	25
Groundnuts	100
Fruit, fresh	200
Fruit, dry	50
Meat	250
Milk, fresh	0.5 litre
Sugar	60
Oil (red palm)	50
Salt	10

Police training college

Food	Amount (grams/head/day)
Maize (*sembe* or *dona*)	500
Bread	100
Potatoes	250
Meat	100
Vegetables (mixed)	150
Fruit	150
Beans	150
Sugar	60
Milk (sweet condensed)	60
Groundnuts	100
Jam	50
Oil (red palm)	25
Salt	10

242

Health training school

Food	Amount (grams/head/day)
Maize (*sembe* or *dona*)	200
Rice	250
Bread (whole meal)	200
Potatoes	200
Beans	100
Groundnuts	50
Onions	25
Green leaves	50
Vegetables (mixed)	75
Fruit (mixed)	100
Sugar	60
Meat	100
Fish	25
Eggs	30
Butter	25
Milk (full-cream powder)	25
Oil (red palm)	25
Salt	10

Farmer-training centre

Food	Amount (grams/head/day)
Maize (*dona*)	500
Rice	100
Beans	150
Vegetables (mixed)	100
Green leaves	50
Eggs	30
Meat	50
Dried fish (*dagaa*)	50
Groundnuts	75
Sugar	50
Oil (red palm)	25
Salt	10

38. DIETS FOR INDUSTRIAL WORKERS

Industrial and estate workers form the main group of Africans who do not produce food of their own. They therefore pose a nutritional problem that differs from much of the rest of the population. The proper feeding of these workers and their families thus needs special attention.

A midday meal should, if possible, be provided for urban industrial workers. This should either be given free or at highly subsidized prices, and on a credit basis so as to encourage as many workers as possible to partake of it. Canteen meals for workers may be expected to result in a higher output of work, a healthier, more contented labour force, and reduced absenteeism. It is therefore often an economic proposition for an employer to provide such a meal.

The suggestions made below are divided into those concerning snacks, which are cheap, easy to prepare and fairly nutritious; and meals, which are a little more costly, require more preparation, but are highly nutritious. The approximate costs given refer to 1978 conditions.

Snacks

1. GRUEL OR *uji*

Ingredients	Amount (grams/head)
Maize meal	300
Sugar	15
Milk powder (DSM)	15 (or equivalent fresh milk)

Cost: Approx. KSh 0.50 (US$0.06) per head
Contains: 1 000 Calories and 25 g protein

2. SOUP AND BREAD

	Ingredients	Amount (grams/head)
Soup:	Dried peas, beans or lentils	50
	Vegetables (mixed)	50
	Meat	15
	Rice	30
	Onions	10
	Oil	4
	Salt	4
Bread:		50

Cost: Approx. KSh 1 (US$ 0.12) per head
Contains: 445 Calories and 19 g protein

Meals

1. *Ugali* AND STEW

Ingredients	Amount (grams/head)
Maize meal	250
Beans (dried)	30
Meat	50
Vegetables (mixed)	75
Oil	4
Salt	4

Cost: Approx. KSh 1.30 (US$0.15) per head
Contains: 1 000 Calories and 45 g protein

2. RICE, STEW, FRUIT, AND TEA

Ingredients	Amount (grams/head)
Rice	200
Beans	30
Meat	50
Vegetables (mixed)	75
Oil	4
Salt	4
Orange	50
Tea	1
Milk powder	15
Sugar	15

Cost: Approx.: KSh 2 (US$ 0.25) per head
Contains: 1 000 Calories and 40 g protein

39.   HOME PRESERVATION OF FOOD

Most dried cereals and legumes, if well stored, last for long periods with little loss of nutritive value and not much deterioration. Many tubers and roots such as cassava, potatoes and yams can also be stored for a few months but are more liable to spoil if conditions are not good. Most other foods are best eaten fresh.

For a number of reasons fresh foods such as fruit, vegetables, meat and fish may not be available to a householder at all times. This may be because the product is seasonal or it is not obtainable locally or for one of many other reasons. It is then to the family's advantage if some preserved foods are used.

Most fresh animal products such as meat and fish deteriorate very rapidly in hot climates. They usually soften and begin to produce an offensive smell. This process of putrefaction is due mainly to the action of bacteria. Most preservation methods serve to prevent or limit the growth of these bacteria. The main preservation methods used in African households are smoking, drying, and wet and dry salting.

Smoking

This is a common traditional practice for meat and fish (see Fig. 64). Typically, meat is cut into strips about 15 cm in length and 2.5-5 cm in diameter. The strips are placed on a rack made of wood or expanded metal over a slow fire. Smoke passes over the surfaces of the meat.

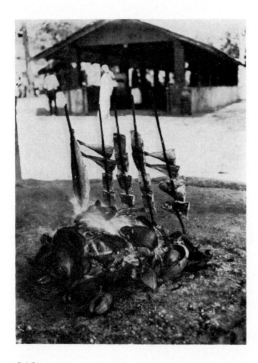

FIGURE 64. Traditional way of smoking fish using coconut shells for fuel.

246

Fish is preserved in the same way after degutting (the guts contain many bacteria).

Drying

Meat, fish, vegetables and fruit can be sun-dried. This method relies on the fact that most bacteria do not readily multiply in a dry medium. When applied to vegetables, it causes some vitamin loss. Sun-drying is especially suitable for small sardine-like fish (e.g., *dagaa*).

Salting

This method is suitable for both meat and fish. It is especially useful for meat, which is not easily preserved by sun-drying. There are a number of salting methods in current use; two simple and suitable ones are the dry and wet methods.

Dry method. Cut the meat into strips as for smoking. Use 300 g of rock or other salt for each 5 kg meat. Roll each meat strip in salt. Use a wooden box or a petrol tin cut in half longitudinally as a container, into which put a layer of salt, a layer of meat, a layer of salt, etc., until full. Leave for 2 days, remove the meat and thread it on string or wire. Hang it in a dry shady part of the house (preferably away from flies). Re-salt it after 3 days. Hang it up again and leave it until the meat is dry and hard (usually 3-4 weeks). The meat will now keep for a long period. It can be eaten either by itself uncooked or it can be used in cooking.

In the latter case it should be cut up and soaked in water for 24 hours. This will serve both to remove some of the salt and to allow it to swell out or rehydrate. It will still taste rather salty, but can be used in soups, stews, and sauces.

Wet method. Cut the meat in strips as above. Use 500 g (1 lb) rock or other salt for each 5 litres (1 gallon) of water. A thoroughly clean 20-litre (4-gallon) petrol tin is a suitable container. If the tin is half filled with water, then 1 kg (2 lb) of rock salt can be added and stirred vigorously. The meat is immersed in the salt water, and left for 3 days. It must remain below the surface. This can be achieved by placing the previously cut out square top of the tin on the surface of the water with a stone on it to add pressure. The meat should be removed after 3 days. It is then hung up and dried as in the above method.

247

A combination of salting and smoking is sometimes used, especially for the preservation of fish.

Fruit preservation with sugar

Like salt, sugar will prevent bacterial growth. However, it is usually more expensive than salt, and larger quantities are required. For every 5 kg fruit (after removal of skin and pips), 3 kg sugar should be used. The fruit and sugar are placed in a cooking pot. Enough water is added to cover the fruit. The pot is simmered on a slow fire for 1 hour. The mixture is removed and put into a container for storage.

Other methods

There are many other methods of food preservation including refrigeration (freezing arrests bacterial growth), canning, bottling, and many chemical processes, which are not suitable for the average African household and are therefore not discussed here.

RECOMMENDED INTAKES OF NUTRIENTS

Table 1 in this appendix forms the basis on which advice can be given regarding recommended intakes of nutrients in diets for particular groups of people in Africa. It also serves as a standard by which to gauge the adequacy of institutional or family diets: after ascertaining the quantity of each food consumed, Appendix 3 can be consulted for the nutritional content of each food; the totals are added and the result can then be compared with the recommended allowances.

This table of recommended intake of nutrients, like similar tables for specific countries, applies to groups of persons and not to individuals. It does not take account of the high rate of parasitic infection that exists in much of Africa. The recommended intakes of iron should be increased by 4-10 mg per day in areas where iron loss due to hookworm disease or other causes is common.

These allowances, in normal circumstances, provide sufficient of each nutrient to prevent deficiency diseases and to allow growth and healthy maintenance of the body at optimum weight and activity.

TABLE 1. RECOMMENDED DAILY INTAKE OF NUTRIENTS FOR POPULATIONS IN AFRICA

Population group	Energy (Calories)	Protein [1] (g)	Calcium (g)	Iron [2] (mg)	Vitamin A [3] (μg)	Thiamine (mg)	Riboflavin (mg)	Niacin (mg)	Vitamin C (mg)
Adult man (55 kg)									
Sedentary	2 310	31	0.4-0.5	5-9	750	0.9	1.4	15.3	30
Active	2 530	31	0.4-0.5	5-9	750	1.0	1.5	16.7	30
Very active	2 970	31	0.4-0.5	5-9	750	1.2	1.8	19.6	30
Adult woman (47 kg)									
Sedentary	1 690	24	0.4-0.5	14-28	750	0.7	1.0	11.2	30
Active	1 880	24	0.4-0.5	14-28	750	0.8	1.1	12.4	30
Very active	2 210	24	0.4-0.5	14-28	750	0.9	1.3	14.6	30
Pregnant (second half of pregnancy)	+350	33	1.0-1.2	14-28	750	+0.1	+0.2	+2.3	50
Lactating (first 6 months of lactation)	+550	41	1.0-1.2	14-28	1 200	+0.2	+0.3	+3.6	50
Adolescents									
Boys: 10-12 years	2 600	30	0.6-0.7	5-10	575	1.0	1.6	17.2	20
13-15 years	2 450	30	0.6-0.7	9-18	725	1.0	1.5	16.2	30
16-19 years	2 580	30	0.5-0.6	5-9	750	1.0	1.6	17.0	30
Girls: 10-12 years	2 350	29	0.6-0.7	5-10	575	0.9	1.4	15.5	20
13-15 years	2 120	29	0.6-0.7	12-24	725	0.9	1.3	14.0	30
16-19 years	1 970	29	0.5-0.6	14-28	750	0.8	1.2	13.0	30
Children:									
Below 1 year	820	14	0.5-0.6	5-10	300	0.3	0.5	5.4	20
1-3 years	1 360	16	0.4-0.5	5-10	250	0.5	0.8	9.0	20
4-6 years	1 830	20	0.4-0.5	5-10	300	0.7	1.1	12.1	20
7-9 years	2 190	25	0.4-0.5	5-10	400	0.9	1.3	14.5	20

Source: FAO, 1974.
[1] As egg or milk protein. — [2] The lower value in the range applies when 25% of the calories in the diet come from animal foods, and the higher value when less than 10% of calories come from this source. — [3] As retinol.

TABLE 2. PER CAPUT DAILY LOCAL ENERGY AND PROTEIN REQUIREMENTS
IN SOME AFRICAN COUNTRIES

Country	Energy (*Calories*)	Protein (*grams*)
Cameroon	2 370	38.1
Ethiopia	2 330	39.9
Ghana	2 300	36.5
Ivory Coast	2 360	35.7
Kenya	2 370	38.8
Mauritius	2 270	36.5
Mozambique	2 340	41.7
Nigeria	2 360	42.9
Senegal	2 385	34.7
Sierra Leone	2 300	38.8
Uganda	2 330	37.3
Zambia	2 310	39.3

Note: The requirements given in FAO/WHO (1973) were determined on the basis of population distribution by sex and age group and requirements per caput per day. The figures for local protein requirement were established by first determining the safe-levels of protein requirements as egg or milk protein and then correcting for the nutritive value of local protein.

DENTITION TABLES AND ANTHROPOMETRIC TABLES

TABLE 1. Average age of dentition

First teeth	Age (*months*)
Central incisors, lower	7 - 8
Central incisors, upper	8 - 9
Lateral incisors, upper	9 - 11
Lateral incisors, lower	10 - 12
First molars	12 - 18
Canines	18 - 24
Second molars	24 - 36

Permanent teeth	Age (*years*)
First molars	6
Central incisors	6 - 7
Lateral incisors	8
Lower canines	10
First premolars	10
Upper canines	11
Second premolars	11
Second molars	12 - 14

TABLE 2. WEIGHT-FOR-AGE, BIRTH TO 60 MONTHS, BOTH SEXES
(*Kilograms*)

Age (months)	Percentage of standard				
	100 (standard)	90	80	70	60
0	3.4	3.0	2.7	2.4	2.0
1	4.3	3.7	3.4	2.9	2.5
2	5.0	4.4	4.0	3.4	2.9
3	5.7	5.1	4.5	4.0	3.4
4	6.3	5.7	5.0	4.5	3.8
5	6.9	6.2	5.5	4.9	4.2
6	7.4	6.7	5.9	5.2	4.5
7	8.0	7.1	6.3	5.5	4.9
8	8.4	7.6	6.7	5.9	5.1
9	8.9	8.0	7.1	6.2	5.3
10	9.3	8.4	7.4	6.5	5.5
11	9.6	8.7	7.7	6.7	5.8
12	9.9	8.9	7.9	6.9	6.0
13	10.2	9.1	8.1	7.1	6.2
14	10.4	9.35	8.3	7.3	6.3
15	10.6	9.5	8.5	7.4	6.4
16	10.8	9.7	8.7	7.6	6.6
17	11.0	9.9	8.9	7.8	6.7
18	11.3	10.1	9.0	7.9	6.8
19	11.5	10.3	9.2	8.1	7.0
20	11.7	10.5	9.4	8.2	7.1
21	11.9	10.7	9.6	8.3	7.2
22	12.05	10.9	9.7	8.4	7.3
23	12.2	11.1	9.8	8.6	7.4
24	12.4	11.2	9.9	8.7	7.5
25	12.6	11.4	10.1	8.9	7.6
26	12.7	11.6	10.3	9.0	7.7
27	12.9	11.8	10.5	9.2	7.8
28	13.1	12.0	10.6	9.3	7.9
29	13.3	12.1	10.7	9.4	8.0
30	13.5	12.2	10.8	9.5	8.1

TABLE 2. WEIGHT-FOR-AGE, BIRTH TO 60 MONTHS, BOTH SEXES (*concluded*)
(*Kilograms*)

Age (months)	Percentage of standard				
	100 (standard)	90	80	70	60
31	13.7	12.4	11.0	9.7	8.2
32	13.8	12.5	11.1	9.8	8.3
33	14.0	12.65	11.2	9.9	8.4
34	14.2	12.8	11.3	10.0	8.5
35	14.4	12.9	11.5	10.1	8.6
36	14.5	13.1	11.6	10.2	8.7
37	14.7	13.2	11.8	10.3	8.8
38	14.85	13.4	11.9	10.4	8.9
39	15.0	13.5	12.05	10.5	9.0
40	15.2	13.6	12.2	10.6	9.1
41	15.35	13.75	12.3	10.7	9.2
42	15.5	13.9	12.4	10.8	9.3
43	15.7	14.0	12.6	10.9	9.4
44	15.85	14.2	12.7	11.05	9.5
45	16.0	14.4	12.9	11.2	9.6
46	16.2	14.6	12.95	11.3	9.7
47	16.35	14.7	13.1	11.4	9.8
48	16.5	14.8	13.2	11.5	9.9
49	16.65	15.0	13.35	11.6	10.0
50	16.8	15.2	13.5	11.75	10.1
51	16.95	15.3	13.65	11.9	10.2
52	17.1	15.45	13.8	12.0	10.3
53	17.25	15.6	13.9	12.1	10.4
54	17.4	15.7	14.0	12.2	10.5
55	17.6	15.85	14.2	12.3	10.6
56	17.7	16.0	14.3	12.4	10.7
57	17.9	16.15	14.4	12.6	10.75
58	18.05	16.3	14.5	12.7	10.8
59	18.25	16.4	14.6	12.8	10.9
60	18.4	16.5	14.7	12.9	11.0

Source: Values derived from Harvard Standards by Stuart and Stevenson (1959).

255

TABLE 3. LENGTH-FOR-AGE, BIRTH TO 60 MONTHS, BOTH SEXES
(*Centimetres*)

Age (months)	Percentage of standard				
	100 (standard)	90	80	70	60
0	50.4	45.4	40.3	35.3	30.2
1	54.8	48.7	43.3	38.3	32.5
2	58.0	51.7	46.2	40.5	34.5
3	60.0	54.0	48.0	42.0	36.0
4	62.3	56.3	49.5	43.3	37.3
5	64.4	58.1	51.1	44.8	38.5
6	65.8	59.2	52.6	46.1	39.5
7	67.6	60.7	54.1	47.2	40.5
8	69.2	62.0	55.3	48.3	41.5
9	70.7	63.6	56.5	49.5	42.4
10	72.2	64.9	57.7	50.4	43.2
11	73.5	66.0	58.8	51.3	44.1
12	74.7	67.2	59.8	52.3	44.8
13	76.0	68.3	60.7	53.1	45.4
14	77.1	69.3	61.6	54.0	46.2
15	78.1	70.3	62.4	54.6	46.8
16	79.3	71.3	63.3	55.4	47.5
17	80.5	72.3	64.2	56.3	48.2
18	81.4	73.2	65.1	57.0	48.8
19	82.7	74.2	65.8	57.7	49.4
20	83.5	75.1	66.9	58.4	50.0
21	84.4	76.0	67.4	59.0	50.7
22	85.4	76.9	68.3	59.7	51.3
23	86.3	77.7	68.9	60.2	51.8
24	87.1	78.4	69.6	60.9	52.2
25	88.0	79.1	70.3	61.2	52.7
26	88.8	80.0	71.0	62.0	53.3
27	89.7	80.7	71.5	62.7	53.8
28	90.4	81.3	72.2	63.2	54.2
29	91.3	82.0	72.8	63.7	54.7
30	91.8	82.6	73.4	64.2	55.1

Age (months)	Percentage of standard				
	100 (standard)	90	80	70	60
31	92.6	83.2	74.0	64.7	55.5
32	93.3	83.7	74.6	65.2	56.0
33	94.0	84.4	75.1	65.7	56.3
34	94.7	85.0	75.7	66.2	56.7
35	95.3	85.7	76.3	66.7	57.2
36	96.0	86.4	76.8	67.2	57.6
37	96.6	87.0	77.3	67.6	58.0
38	97.3	87.5	78.0	68.1	58.3
39	97.9	88.0	78.4	68.6	58.7
40	98.4	88.5	78.9	69.0	59.2
41	99.1	89.1	79.3	69.4	59.5
42	99.7	89.7	79.7	69.8	59.8
43	100.3	90.3	80.2	70.3	60.2
44	101.0	90.9	80.7	70.7	60.5
45	101.6	91.5	81.3	71.1	60.9
46	102.1	92.0	81.7	71.5	61.2
47	102.7	92.6	82.1	72.0	61.7
48	103.3	93.0	82.6	72.3	62.0
49	103.8	93.6	83.2	72.7	62.3
50	104.5	94.0	83.6	73.1	62.7
51	105.2	94.5	84.0	73.4	63.1
52	105.7	95.1	84.4	73.8	63.5
53	106.2	95.6	84.9	74.3	63.8
54	106.8	96.1	85.4	74.7	64.1
55	107.3	96.5	85.7	75.0	64.4
56	107.9	96.8	86.0	75.3	64.7
57	108.2	97.2	86.3	75.7	64.9
58	108.5	97.5	86.7	75.9	65.1
59	108.7	97.7	86.9	76.1	65.2
60	109.0	98.0	87.1	76.2	65.3

Source: Values derived from Harvard Standards by Stuart and Stevenson (1959).

TABLE 4. WEIGHT-FOR-LENGTH, YOUNG CHILDREN, BOTH SEXES
(*Kilograms*)

Length (cm)	Percentage of standard				
	100 (standard)	90	80	70	60
52	3.8	3.4	3.0	2.7	2.3
53	4.0	3.6	3.2	2.8	2.4
54	4.3	3.9	3.4	3.0	2.6
55	4.6	4.1	3.6	3.2	2.7
56	4.8	4.3	3.8	3.4	2.9
57	5.0	4.5	3.9	3.5	3.0
58	5.2	4.7	4.2	3.6	3.1
59	5.5	4.9	4.4	3.8	3.3
60	5.7	5.1	4.6	4.0	3.4
61	6.0	5.4	4.8	4.2	3.6
62	6.3	5.7	5.0	4.4	3.8
63	6.6	5.9	5.3	4.6	3.9
64	6.9	6.2	5.5	4.8	4.1
65	7.2	6.5	5.8	5.0	4.3
66	7.5	6.8	6.0	5.3	4.5
67	7.8	7.0	6.2	5.5	4.7
68	8.1	7.3	6.5	5.7	4.9
69	8.4	7.6	6.7	5.9	5.0
70	8.7	7.8	7.0	6.1	5.2
71	9.0	8.1	7.2	6.2	5.3
72	9.2	8.3	7.4	6.4	5.5
73	9.5	8.5	7.6	6.6	5.6
74	9.7	8.7	7.8	6.8	5.8
75	9.9	9.0	8.0	6.9	5.9
76	10.2	9.2	8.3	7.1	6.1
77	10.4	9.4	8.3	7.2	6.2
78	10.6	9.5	8.5	7.4	6.4
79	10.8	9.7	8.6	7.5	6.5
80	11.0	9.9	8.8	7.7	6.6
81	11.2	10.1	9.0	7.8	6.7
82	11.4	10.3	9.1	8.0	6.8

TABLE 4. WEIGHT-FOR-LENGTH, YOUNG CHILDREN, BOTH SEXES (*concluded*)
(*Kilograms*)

Length (cm)	Percentage of standard				
	100 (standard)	90	80	70	60
83	11.6	10.4	9.2	8.1	6.9
84	11.8	10.6	9.4	8.3	7.1
85	12.0	10.7	9.6	8.4	7.2
86	12.2	11.0	9.8	8.5	7.3
87	12.4	11.1	9.9	8.6	7.4
88	12.6	11.3	10.1	8.8	7.6
89	12.8	11.5	10.2	9.0	7.7
90	13.1	11.8	10.5	9.2	7.9
91	13.4	11.9	10.7	9.3	8.0
92	13.6	12.2	10.9	9.5	8.2
93	13.8	12.4	11.0	9.6	8.3
94	14.0	12.6	11.2	9.8	8.4
95	14.3	12.8	11.4	10.0	8.5
96	14.5	13.1	11.6	10.2	8.7
97	14.7	13.3	11.8	10.3	8.8
98	15.0	13.5	12.0	10.5	9.0
99	15.3	13.7	12.3	10.7	9.2
100	15.6	14.0	12.5	10.9	9.4
101	15.8	14.2	12.6	11.1	9.5
102	16.1	14.5	12.9	11.3	9.7
103	16.4	14.7	13.2	11.5	9.8
104	16.7	15.0	13.4	11.7	10.0
105	17.0	15.3	13.6	11.9	10.1
106	17.3	15.6	13.8	12.1	10.4
107	17.6	15.7	14.0	12.3	10.5
108	18.0	16.2	14.4	12.6	10.8

Source: Values derived from Harvard Standards by Stuart and Stevenson (1959).

TABLE 5. ARM CIRCUMFERENCE, 1-60 MONTHS, BY SEX
(Centimetres)

Age (months)	Percentage of standard					
	100 (standard)		80		60	
	M	F	M	F	M	F
1	11.5	11.1	9.2	8.9	6.9	6.7
2	12.5	12.0	10.0	9.6	7.5	7.2
3	12.7	13.3	10.2	10.6	7.6	8.0
4	14.6	13.5	11.7	10.8	8.8	8.1
5	14.7	13.9	11.7	11.1	8.8	8.3
6	14.5	14.3	11.6	11.5	8.7	8.6
7	15.0	14.6	12.0	11.7	9.0	8.8
8	15.5	15.0	12.4	12.0	9.3	9.0
9	15.8	15.3	12.6	12.2	9.5	9.2
10	15.8	15.4	12.6	12.3	9.5	9.2
11	15.8	15.5	12.7	12.4	9.5	9.3
12	16.0	15.6	12.8	12.5	9.6	9.4
15	16.1	15.7	12.9	12.5	9.7	9.4
18	15.7	16.1	12.5	12.9	9.4	9.7
21	16.2	15.9	13.0	12.7	9.7	9.6
24	16.3	15.9	13.0	12.8	9.8	9.6
27	16.6	16.4	13.3	13.1	10.0	9.8
30	16.4	16.4	13.1	13.1	9.9	9.8
33	16.4	16.1	13.1	12.9	9.8	9.7
36	16.2	15.9	13.0	12.7	9.7	9.6
39	16.9	17.4	13.5	14.0	10.1	10.5
42	16.5	16.3	13.2	13.1	9.9	9.8
45	16.7	16.8	13.4	13.5	10.0	10.1
48	16.9	16.9	13.5	13.5	10.1	10.2
51	17.2	16.8	13.8	13.4	10.3	10.1
54	17.5	16.6	14.0	13.3	10.5	10.0
57	17.2	16.8	13.8	13.4	10.4	10.1
60	17.0	16.9	13.6	13.5	10.2	10.1

Source: WHO, 1966.
Note: M = Male; F = Female.

TABLE 6. STANDARD TRICEPS SKINFOLD, BIRTH TO 60 MONTHS, BY SEX
(*Millimetres*)

Age (months)	Male	Female
0	6.0	6.5
6	10.0	10.0
12	10.3	10.2
18	10.3	10.2
24	10.0	10.1
36	9.3	9.7
48	9.3	10.2
60	9.1	9.4

Source: WHO, 1966.

TABLE 7. STANDARD TRICEPS SKINFOLD, 5-15 YEARS, BY SEX
(*Millimetres*)

Age (years)	Male	Female
5	9.1	9.4
6	8.2	9.6
7	7.9	9.4
8	7.6	10.1
9	8.2	10.3
10	8.2	10.4
11	8.9	10.6
12	8.5	10.1
13	8.1	10.4
14	7.9	11.3
15	6.3	11.4

Source: WHO, 1966.

TABLE 8. STANDARD ARM CIRCUMFERENCE, 6-17 YEARS, BY SEX
(*Centimetres*)

Age (years)	Male	Female
6	17.3	17.3
7	17.8	17.8
8	18.4	18.4
9	19.0	19.1
10	19.7	19.9
11	20.4	20.7
12	21.2	21.5
13	22.2	23.2
14	23.2	23.2
15	25.0	24.4
16	26.0	24.7
17	26.8	24.9

Source: WHO, 1966.

TABLE 9. TRICEPS SKINFOLD, ADULTS, BY SEX
(*Millimetres*)

Sex	Percentage of standard				
	100 (standard)	90	80	70	60
Male	12.5	11.3	10.0	8.8	7.5
Female	16.5	14.9	13.2	11.6	9.9

Source: WHO, 1966.

TABLE 10. ARM CIRCUMFERENCE, ADULTS, BY SEX
(*Centimetres*)

Sex	Percentage of standard				
	100 (standard)	90	80	70	60
Male	29.3	26.3	23.4	20.5	17.6
Female	28.5	25.7	22.8	20.0	17.1

Source: WHO, 1966.

262

NUTRITIONAL CONTENT OF TYPICAL AFRICAN FOODS

NUTRITIONAL CONTENT OF TYPICAL AFRICAN FOODS

(*Per 100 grams of edible portion*)

Cereals

Item No.	Foods	Water ml	Energy Calories	Protein g	Fat g	Carbohydrate g	Fibre g	Calcium mg	Iron mg	Vitamins						Waste (% of food as purchased)
										Retinol µg	β-carotene equiv. µg	Thiamine mg	Riboflavin mg	Niacin mg	Ascorbic acid mg	
1	Maize, whole grain	11	359	9.3	4.4	73.7	1.8	12	3.8	...	[1]41	0.34	0.10	1.8	3	[2]0
2	Maize meal, about 96% extraction	12	362	9.5	4.0	72.0	1.5	12	2.5	...	[1]tr	0.30	0.13	1.5	0	0
3	Maize meal, refined, 60% extraction	12	354	8.0	1.5	77.0	0.7	9	2.0	...	[1]tr	0.05	0.03	0.6	0	0
4	Millet, bulrush, whole grains	12	341	10.4	4.0	71.6	1.9	22	20.7	...	tr	0.30	0.22	1.7	3	0
5	Millet, finger, whole grain	11	329	7.4	1.3	77.7	4.3	397	17.1	...	tr	0.18	0.11	0.8	0	0
6	Rice, lightly milled and parboiled	12	364	7.0	0.6	79.8	0.4	6	2.4	...	tr	0.17	0.03	5.4	0	0
7	Rice, highly milled, polished	12	363	7.0	0.5	79.9	0.4	9	1.7	...	0	0.10	0.03	2.8	0	0
8	Sorghum, whole															

Starchy roots, tubers and fruits

10	Wheat, whole grain	12	332	12.7	1.8	71.8	2.6	60	7.6	...	0	0.35	0.12	3.6	0	0
11	Wheat flour, 85% extraction	12	351	10.5	2.0	74.7	0.8	36	3.6	...	tr	0.37	0.08	2.8	0	0
12	Wheat flour, 72% extraction	12	364	10.3	1.0	76.2	0.2	27	2.2	...	0	0.08	0.05	0.8	0	0
13	Cassava, fresh (*Manihot*)	62	149	1.2	0.2	35.7	1.1	68	1.9	...	30	0.04	0.05	0.6	31	[3] 26
14	Cassava flour	9	363	1.1	0.5	88.2	2.2	84	1.0	...	tr	0.02	0.03	0.6	0	0
15	Plantain	65	135	1.2	0.3	32.1	0.5	8	1.3	...	780	0.08	0.04	0.6	20	34
16	Potato, Irish	78	82	1.7	0.1	18.9	0.6	13	1.1	...	25	0.07	0.03	1.3	[4] 21	14
17	Potato, sweet	69	121	1.6	0.2	28.5	1.0	33	2.0	...	75	0.09	0.04	0.7	37	21
18	Taro	73	102	1.8	0.1	23.8	1.0	51	1.2	...	tr	0.10	0.03	0.8	8	16
19	Taro, giant and other starchy aroids	70	111	0.5	tr	27.0	1.2	150	1.0	...	tr	0.03	0.10	1.0	tr	...
20	Yam, fresh	69	119	1.9	0.2	27.8	0.8	52	0.8	...	10	0.11	0.02	0.3	6	[5] 16
21	Yam flour	14	335	3.4	0.4	80.0	1.6	20	1.1	...	tr	0.10	0.08	1.1	0	0

Sources: FAO (1968), and Platt (1962).

NOTE: ... = data not available

tr = trace, contains too small a quantity to be significant in dietary evaluations

[1] Yellow maize, 90 µg β-carotene equivalent, range 60-360 µg.
[2] For ripe maize on cob with sheath, waste is 25 percent.
[3] If thin outer peel is removed only after cooking, waste is 5 percent.
[4] Decreases during storage.
[5] For larger varieties waste may be as low as 5 percent.

265

NUTRITIONAL CONTENT OF TYPICAL AFRICAN FOODS

(Per 100 grams of edible portion)

(continued)

Item No.	Foods	Water ml	Energy Calories	Protein g	Fat g	Carbohydrate g	Fibre g	Calcium mg	Iron mg	Retinol μg	β-carotene equiv. μg	Vitamins				Waste (% of food as purchased)
												Thiamine mg	Riboflavin mg	Niacin mg	Ascorbic acid mg	
Grain legumes and products																
22	Bambara groundnut	10	367	18.8	6.2	61.3	4.8	62	12.2	...	10	0.47	0.14	1.8	tr	25
23	Chick-pea	10	357	19.6	3.7	63.5	6.7	252	11.1	...	60	0.48	0.16	1.8	tr	0
24	Cowpea	11	338	22.5	1.4	61.0	5.4	104	7.6	...	12	0.08	0.09	4.0	2	0
25	Groundnut, dry	7	549	23.2	44.8	23.0	2.9	49	3.8	...	15	0.79	0.14	15.5	1	30
26	Groundnut, fresh	45	332	15.0	25.0	12.0	1.5	30	1.5	...	tr	0.50	0.10	10.0	10	35
27	Horse gram	10	333	22.5	1.0	60.5	4.7	280	8.0	...	24	0.40	0.15	2.5	tr	...
28	Kidney bean	12	336	21.7	1.5	60.9	4.4	120	8.2	...	10	0.37	0.16	2.4	1	0
29	Lathyrus pea	8	348	27.4	1.1	59.8	7.3	127	10.0	...	42	0.10	0.40	...	tr	...
30	Lentil	10	345	24.9	1.2	61.1	3.9	64	7.0	...	60	0.41	0.19	2.2	tr	0
31	Pea	11	339	22.3	1.1	62.0	5.7	90	17.9	...	15	0.88	0.17	3.0	tr	0
32	Pigeon pea	10	345	19.5	1.3	65.5	7.3	161	15.0	...	55	0.72	0.14	2.9	tr	0
33	Scarlet runner bean	13	338	20.3	1.8	62.0	4.8	114	9.0	...	tr	0.50	0.19	2.3	2	0
34	Soybean seed	10	405	33.7	17.9	33.9	4.7	183	6.1	...	55	0.71	0.25	2.0	tr	0

No.	Food	%	kcal	g	g	g	g	mg	mg		i.u.	mg	mg	mg	mg	mg
36	Cashew nut	8	542	17.4	43.4	29.2	1.4	76	18.0	...	tr	0.65	0.25	1.6	7	...
37	Coconut, kernel, mature, fresh	43	388	3.6	39.0	13.8	6.6	21	2.5	...	tr	0.03	0.03	0.6	2	[6]35
38	Coconut milk, ripe nut	96	14	0.2	tr	3	tr	15	tr	...	tr	tr	tr	tr	1	[7]...
39	Melon seeds, seed coat removed	6	567	25.8	49.7	15.1	4.0	53	7.4	...	tr	0.10	0.12	1.4	tr	25
40	Pumpkin seeds, seed coat removed	6	555	23.4	46.2	21.5	2.2	57	2.8	...	30	0.15	0.20	1.4	2	25
41	Sesame seeds	5	558	17.9	48.4	22.3	4.5	816	8.1	...	30	0.68	0.19	3.4	2	0
42	Sunflower seeds, seed coat removed	6	486	13.0	27.7	51.3	25.9	100	7.0	...	tr	1.90	0.20	5.8	...	50

Vegetables

No.	Food	%	kcal	g	g	g	g	mg	mg		i.u.	mg	mg	mg	mg	mg
43	Beans, eaten green in pod	89	36	2.5	0.2	7.9	1.8	43	1.4	...	750	0.08	0.12	0.5	27	8
44	Beans and peas, fresh shelled	70	104	7.0	tr	19	2.5	40	2.0	...	90	0.30	0.15	1.5	25	55
45	Carrots	89	40	0.9	0.1	9.6	1.4	35	0.7	...	5 480	0.04	0.04	0.6	8	26
46	Cauliflower	92	25	2.0	0.1	5.4	1.2	35	1.2	...	15	0.06	0.09	0.5	96	44
47	Cucumber	95	15	0.8	0.1	3.4	0.8	13	0.5	...	tr	0.02	0.01	0.3	14	28
48	Egg-plant	91	32	1.0	0.2	7.7	1.3	14	1.3	...	34	0.05	0.05	0.5	9	22
49	Gourd (fruit pulp)	94	21	0.5	0.1	5.2	0.6	44	2.4	...	25	0.03	0.03	0.4	10	25

[6] For kernel and milk together, waste is about 20 percent, i.e., kernel averages about 65 percent of ripe nut as purchased.
[7] For kernel and milk together, waste is about 20 percent, i.e., kernel averages about 65 percent and milk 15 percent of ripe nut as purchased.

(Per 100 grams of edible portion)

(continued)

Item No.	Foods	Water ml	Energy Calories	Protein g	Fat g	Carbohydrate g	Fibre g	Calcium mg	Iron mg	Retinol μg	β-carotene equiv. μg	Thiamine mg	Riboflavin mg	Niacin mg	Ascorbic acid mg	Waste (% of food as purchased)
												Vitamins				
	Vegetables (concluded)															
50	Leaves, high carotene, e.g., amaranth	94	42	4.6	0.2	8.3	1.8	410	8.9	...	5 716	0.05	0.42	1.2	64	[8] 24
51	Leaves, medium carotene, e.g., pumpkin	89	27	4.0	0.2	4.4	2.4	477	0.8	...	3 600	0.08	0.06	0.3	80	[8] 20
52	Leaves, low carotene, pale green, e.g., cabbage, kohlrabi, Chinese cabbage, etc.	91	25	2.0	0.3	5.0	1.4	58	0	...	2 280	0	0.18	0.3	40	20
53	Lettuce	94	20	1.2	0.2	4.3	0.6	26	0.7	...	180	0.10	0.10	0.4	10	30
54	Maize, immature ears	58	152	5.0	2.1	34.4	0.8	18	1.8	...	tr	0.16	0.08	1.3	10	30
55	Onion and shallot	89	41	1.2	0.1	9.6	1.0	27	0.8	...	0	0.02	0.04	0.2	11	6
56	Peppers, sweet, green seeds removed	86	48	2.0	0.8	10.3	2.6	29	2.6	...	[9] 180	0.12	0.15	2.2	140	[10] 16

58	Fungi, mixed, fresh	90	11	2.0	0.3	...	1.0	5	1.2	...	tr	0.02	0.40	1.0	tr	9
59	Mushrooms, fresh	[11]91	13	2.5	0.3	...	1.0	20	1.0	...	0	0.12	0.50	5.8	3.0	9
60	Yeast, baker's compressed	71	86	12.1	0.4	11.0	0.5	13	4.9	...	tr	0.71	1.65	11.2	tr	0
61	Yeast, brewer's dry	5	214	50.0	1.5	[12]0	0.5	80	20.0	...	0	9.5	4.0	36.0	0	0

Fruits

62	Apple	34	58	0.2	0.4	15.1	0.8	3	0.2	...	80	0.04	0.02	0.2	1	16
63	Avocado pear	80	121	1.4	11.3	6.1	1.8	19	1.4	...	530	0.05	0.15	2.0	18	50
64	Banana	77	88	1.5	0.1	20.6	0.9	9	1.4	...	120	0.03	0.03	6.0	9	32
65	Cape gooseberry	85	53	1.9	0.7	11.2	9.8	9	1.0	...	430	0.11	0.04	2.8	11	8
66	Citrus, grapefruit, pomelo, etc.	90	34	0.8	0.1	8.6	0.6	21	0.6	...	25	0.05	0.03	0.2	44	49
67	Citrus, lemon and lime	90	32	0.6	0.8	8.7	0.7	19	0.7	...	10	0.03	0.02	0.3	45	41
68	Citrus, orange and tangerine	86	49	0.8	0.3	12.3	0.6	38	1.1	...	230	0.08	0.05	0.2	[13]46	30
69	Dates, dried	17	293	2.7	0.6	77.6	3.9	82	9.4	...	30	0.06	0.15	1.8	tr	13
70	Fig, fresh	85	52	0.8	0.2	13.2	1.3	44	0.5	...	30	0.05	0.05	0.4	15	14

[8] For 16 kinds of leaves used in Malawi, waste varied from 0-60 percent.
[9] For mature, red peppers, the value is about 2 760 µg/100 g.
[10] Seeds, cores and stem ends.
[11] Water content of dried mushrooms, 12 percent.
[12] Carbohydrate not available; cell walls resistant to digestion.
[13] Tangerine, 30 (13-50) mg.

Nutritional content of typical African foods

(Per 100 grams of edible portion)

Item No.	Foods	Water ml	Energy Calories	Protein g	Fat g	Carbohydrate g	Fibre g	Calcium mg	Iron mg	Vitamins						Waste (% of food as purchased)
										Retinol µg	β-carotene equiv. µg	Thiamine mg	Riboflavin mg	Niacin mg	Ascorbic acid mg	

Fruits (concluded)

Item No.	Foods	Water ml	Energy Calories	Protein g	Fat g	Carbohydrate g	Fibre g	Calcium mg	Iron mg	Retinol µg	β-carotene equiv. µg	Thiamine mg	Riboflavin mg	Niacin mg	Ascorbic acid mg	Waste
71	Grenadilla, flesh and seeds	75	92	2.3	14 2.0	16.0	3.5	10	1.0	...	12	tr	0.10	1.5	20	43
72	Guava, flesh and seeds	82	64	1.1	0.4	15.7	5.3	24	1.3	...	290	0.06	0.04	1.3	326	19
73	Mango	83	60	0.6	0.2	15.8	0.9	25	1.2	...	3 200	0.03	0.05	0.4	42	36
74	Melon, sweet	95	18	0.5	0.1	4.2	0.5	20	1.7	...	30	0.04	0.02	0.6	12	20
75	Melon, water	94	23	0.4	tr	5	0.1	5	0.3	...	18	0.02	0.02	0.2	5	50
76	Palm fruit, peach palm, pejibaye	50	209	2.5	3.5	42	1.1	20	1.5	...	300	0.04	0.10	1.5	25	...
77	Papaya	91	32	0.4	0.1	8.3	0.9	21	0.6	...	950	0.03	0.03	0.4	52	26
78	Pineapple	87	47	0.4	0.1	12.4	0.5	16	0.4	...	90	0.06	0.03	0.1	34	33
79	Plum	86	49	0.6	0.2	12.5	1.1	10	0.6	...	770	0.02	0.05	0.3	5	7
80	Pomegranate, raw	78	78	1.6	0.3	19.6	4.5	12	1.0	...	40	0.02	0.03	0.2	8	44
81	Prickly pear, pulp and small seeds	83	62	1.0	0.4	15.4	3.9	31	0.3	...	tr	0.03	0.03	0.3	20	45
82	West Indian cherry	92	31	0.4	0.3	7.0	0.4	12	0.5	...	12	0.03	0.05	0.4	2 000	17

No.	Item														
83	Butter	[15] 21	685	0	77.3	1.5	0	15	0.2	640	545	0	0	0	0	0
84	Fish-liver oils	0	900	0	100.0	0	0	0	0	27 000	[16] 6 000	0	0	0	0	0
85	Ghee	1.4	862	0	97.8	0.6	0	tr	0.4	420	360	0	0	0	0	0
86	Lard and other animal fats	0	902	0	100.0	0	0	0	0	0	0	0	0	0	0	0
87	Margarine	14.0	765	0	85.0	0	0	4	0	...	[17] 1 800	tr	tr	tr	tr	0
88	Red palm oil	0	900	0	100.0	0	0	0	0	...	[18] 12 000	0	0	0	0	0
89	Vegetable oils	0	884	0	110.0	0	0	0	0	...	tr	0	0	0	0	0

Fish and fish products (including molluscs and crustaceans)

No.	Item														
90	Fish, freshwater, fillet	75	119	21.6	3.0	0	0	32	1.7	...	[19] tr	0.05	0.08	2.8	0	48
91	Fish, sea, lean fillet	81	73	17.0	0.5	tr	...	20	0.7	...	tr	0.05	0.10	2.5	tr	0
92	Fish, sea, fillet	70	166	19.0	[20] 10.0	tr	...	30	1.5	27	[21] 6	0.05	0.2	[22] 3.0	tr	0
93	Fish, dried [23]	20	309	63.0	6.3	tr	...	3 000	8.5	...	tr	0.10	0.20	6.0	0	0
94	Crustaceans (lobster, crab, prawns, etc.)	77	94	18.0	1.5	1.5	2	100	5.0	...	tr	0.05	0.10	2.5	tr	63

14 Fat in seed.
15 International Standard: maximum water content 16-20 percent.
16 For cod-liver oil. Halibut-liver oil, average: 2 700 000 µg retinol; 600 000 µg β-carotene. Range: 540 000-9 720 000 µg retinol, 120 000-2 160 000 µg β-carotene.
17 Vitamin A added artificially. Unfortified margarine contains no vitamin A.
18 Values for refined palm oil are lower.
19 Carp are reported to have 46 µg retinol, 10 µg carotene equivalent.
20 Oil content of fat fish varies considerably (usually inversely with water content) according to type of fish, season, locality; e.g., mackerel, 3.9-19.2; herring, 2.6-12.5; salmon 5-16 percent.
21 Vitamin A varies according to species and season.
22 Mackerel, salmon and tuna have higher values for niacin averaging 7.0 mg.
23 Dried freshwater fish with edible bones has been taken as a representative sample.

271

NUTRITIONAL CONTENT OF TYPICAL AFRICAN FOODS

(Per 100 grams of edible portion)

Item No.	Foods	Water ml	Energy Calories	Protein g	Fat g	Carbohydrate g	Fibre g	Calcium mg	Iron mg	Retinol μg	β-carotene equiv. μg	Thiamine mg	Riboflavin mg	Niacin mg	Ascorbic acid mg	Waste (% of food as purchased)
	Fish and fish products (including molluscs and crustaceans) [*concluded*]															
95	Molluscs (oysters, mussels, clams, etc.)	83	70	10.0	2.0	3	...	150	10.0	54	12	0.05	0.15	1.5	tr	75
96	Sardines, canned in oil	50	309	20.0	25.0	1	...	400	3.0	54	12	tr	0.20	4.0	0	0
97	Sea slug (bêche de mer), soaked	76	94	22.0	tr	1	...	120	1.4	...	...	...	...	...	...	0
98	Snail, river, pond	78	82	12.0	2.0	4	...	1 500	8.0	...	...	tr	0.05	1.3	...	53
	Insects and larvae															
99	Lake fly	16	382	48.6	10.3	21.2	(Chitin) 3.4	140	65.6	...	...	1.24	3.44	18.3	...	...
100	Larvae (dried caterpillars, etc.)	[24] 9	430	52.9	15.4	16.9	5.4	185	2.3	220	50	0.17	1.30	6.0	0	...
101	Locusts, mature	[25] 70	134	20.0	6.0	tr	4.0	30	1.0	...	...	...	0.50	2.2	...	...
102	Termites, white ants, mature	75	148	10.0	12.0	tr	1.2	12	1.0	...	...	...	...	...	...	...

No.	Food															
103	Beef, moderately fat, whole carcass	63	237	18.2	17.7	0	0	11	3.6	...	tr	0.07	0.15	4.5	tr	20
104	Beef, lean	75	122	20.6	3.8	0	0	22	4.6	0	tr	0.06	0.17	3.2	0	23
105	Beef, canned, corned	54	251	27.2	15.0	0	0	15	4.0	...	tr	0	0.20	3.5	0	0
106	Eggs, hen and duck	[26] 77	140	11.8	[26] 9.6	0.6	0	45	2.6	350	300	0.12	0.35	0.3	tr	12
107	Goat, carcass	73	145	16.0	9.0	tr	...	11	2.5	...	tr	0.20	0.35	5.0	tr	26
108	Mutton (fat, whole carcass), unspecified	61	265	16.9	21.4	0	0	10	2.0	10	tr	0.15	0.20	3.1	4.5	tr
109	Mutton, moderately fat, whole carcass	63	249	15.0	21.0	tr	...	10	2.4	...	tr	0.15	0.20	4.5	tr	20
110	Mutton, lean, whole carcass	73	149	17.0	9.0	tr	...	11	2.5	...	tr	2.20	0.25	5.0	tr	26
111	Offal, heart	75	129	16.5	7.0	tr	...	10	4.5	54	12	0.60	0.90	7.0	0	...
112	Offal, kidney	75	127	16.0	7.0	tr	...	10	10.0	270	60	0.30	2.00	7.0	[27] 12.0	...
113	Offal, liver	70	136	20.0	4.0	5	...	10	10.0	5 400	[28] 1 200	0.30	2.50	13.0	[27] 30.0	...
114	Pork, fat, whole carcass, medium fat	46	418	12.4	40.5	0	0	11	1.8	...	tr	0.50	0.15	3.0	tr	13
115	Pork, lean, whole carcass	50	371	14.0	35.0	tr	...	10	2.0	...	tr	0.80	0.20	4.0	tr	18

[24] When fresh, water content is 75-85 percent.
[25] When sun-dried, water content is 5 percent.
[26] Duck eggs have 14.5 percent fat and less water than hen eggs.
[27] When fresh.
[28] Variations are very large, both between species and between individuals of the same species: calf and pig are generally lowest (1 350-5 460 μg retinol, 300-1 200 μg β-carotene) and sheep highest (13 500 μg retinol, 3 000 μg β-carotene).

NUTRITIONAL CONTENT OF TYPICAL AFRICAN FOODS

(Per 100 grams of edible portion)

Item No.	Foods	Water ml	Energy Calories	Protein g	Fat g	Carbohydrate g	Fibre g	Calcium mg	Iron mg	Vitamins						Waste (% of food as purchased)
										Retinol μg	β-carotene equiv. μg	Thiamine mg	Riboflavin mg	Niacin mg	Ascorbic acid mg	
Meat, meat products and eggs (concluded)																
116	Pork, salt, fat	8	781	4.0	85.0	0	...	tr	0.6	...	0	0.18	0.04	0.9	0	4
117	Poultry: chicken, duck, turkey, etc.	73	139	19.0	7.0	tr	...	15	1.5	...	tr	0.10	0.15	9.0	tr	33
118	Rabbit	72	134	20.0	6.0	tr	...	15	1.5	...	tr	0.05	0.10	9.0	0	18
Milk and milk products																
119	Cheese from whole cow's milk, hard	39	384	24.0	32.0	tr	...	800	0.5	290	252	0.04	0.50	0.1	0	0
120	Cheese from skim cow's milk, soft	77	87	19.5	0.5	1.0	...	90	0.4	3	3	0.02	0.30	0.1	0	0
121	Milk, cow, whole	[29] 85	79	3.8	[29] 4.8	5.4	0	143	0.2	95	[30] 80	0.04	0.30	0.1	1	0
122	Milk, human	87	67	1.1	3.1	9.1	0	30	0.2	33	28	0.02	0.04	0.2	4	0
123	Milk, goat	84	85	3.4	4.9	7.0	0	130	0.1	25	22	0.05	0.10	0.3	1	0
124	Milk, sheep	83	100	5.9	7.0	3.5	0	200	0.1	54	12	0.07	0.50	0.5	2	0
125	Milk, cow,															

No.		Water (g)	Energy (kcal)	Protein (g)	Fat (g)	Carbohydrate (g)	Fibre (g)	Ca (mg)	Fe (mg)							
126	Milk, cow, whole, condensed	[31] 74	140	7.0	8.0	10.0	0	260	0.2	67	[30] 58	0.06	0.32	0.21	1.7	0
127	Milk, cow, whole, condensed, sweetened	29	317	7.3	8.0	53.9	0	270	0.2	74	[30] 63	0.09	0.33	0.20	3.8	0
128	Milk, cow, whole, powder	4	500	25.5	27.5	37.5	0	900	0.8	252	[30] 216	0.30	1.15	0.76	13.0	0
129	Milk, cow, skim, condensed, sweetened	29	276	9.6	0.3	58.8	0	340	0.3	3	2	0.12	0.40	0.30	4.8	0
130	Milk, cow, skim, powder	4	357	36.0	1.0	51.0	0	1 260	1.0	8	5	0.45	1.53	1.1	17.0	0
	Condiments and spices															
131	Chilies, hot, dried	13	312	13.9	9.4	56.0	11.1	538	9.0	…	[32] 1 060	0	0.20	4.4	10	…
132	Cloves, dried flower buds	23	293	5.0	9.0	48.0	10.0	740	5.0	…	…	0.10	0.20	2.0	0	…
133	Garlic	63	131	5.2	0.1	30.2	1.0	33	1.7	…	tr	0.25	0.08	0.4	11	…
	Syrups, sugars and preserves															
134	Honey	23	286	0.4	tr	[33] 76	0	5	0.4	…	tr	tr	0.05	0.2	tr	0
135	Jam [34]	29	260	0.4	tr	[33] 69	0.6	12	0.3	…	tr	tr	tr	tr	[35] 10	0

29 In very hot climates water is less, as low as 84 percent, and fat is higher, up to 6.2 percent.
30 Varies according to season and feedstuffs.
31 There are two different degrees of concentration on the international market. The one given is used in the US and currently in the UK.
32 Red varieties have the higher value.
33 Expressed as monosaccharide; conversion factor for calculating Calories: 3.75.
34 Average values for jam prepared from various fruits.
35 According to type of fruit.

NUTRITIONAL CONTENT OF TYPICAL AFRICAN FOODS

(Per 100 grams of edible portion)

Item No.	Foods	Water ml	Energy Calories	Protein g	Fat g	Carbohydrate g	Fibre g	Calcium mg	Iron mg	Retinol μg	β-carotene equiv. μg	Thiamine mg	Riboflavin mg	Niacin mg	Ascorbic acid mg	Waste (% of food as purchased)
										Vitamins						
Syrups, sugars and preserves (concluded)																
136	Sugar, crude brown	8	344	0.2	tr	88.8	0	30	20	...	tr	0.02	0.1	0.3	0	0
137	Sugar-cane juice	81	73	0.3	tr	18.0	tr	6	2.0	...	tr	0.02	0.02	0.1	tr	0
138	Sugar, white	tr	400	0	0	100	0	0	0	0	0	0	0	0	0	0
Miscellaneous																
139	Banana and plantain flowers	91	29	1.4	0.4	5	1.0	4.0	0.3	...	60	0.02	0.03	0.4	1-12	55
140	Maize and sorghum stems	75	58	0.5	tr	14	...	25	1.0	...	0	tr	...	...	tr	...
141	Sugar-cane stems	83	62	0.6	0.1	16.5	[36] 3.1	8	1.4	...	0	0.02	0.01	0.1	3	55

[36] Fibre may be as high as 10-15 percent.

Appendix 4

CONVERSION TABLES

Appendix 5

GLOSSARY OF VERNACULAR WORDS

CONVERSION TABLES [1]

Length

1 centimetre (cm) = 0.4 inches (in.)
1 metre (m) = 100 cm = 39 in. (approx. 3 feet)
1 inch = 2.5 cm
1 foot = 30.5 cm

Weight

100 milligrams (mg) = 1.5 grains (gn)
1 grain = 65 mg
100 grams (g) = 3.6 ounces (oz)
1 ounce = 28.3 g
1 kilogram (kg) = 2.2 pounds (lb)

Fluid measures

1 millilitre (ml) = 17 minims (min)
1 fluid ounce (fl oz) = 30 ml
1 litre (l) = 1.8 pints (pt) = 35.2 fl oz
1 pint = 570 ml
1 teaspoonful = 4 ml = 1/8 fl oz
1 tablespoonful = 15 ml = 1/2 fl oz

Temperature

Temperature in °C = (Temperature in °F — 32) × 5/9
Temperature in °F = Temperature in °C × 9/5 + 32
Freezing point = 0°C = 32°F
Boiling point = 100°C = 212°F

Energy

1 Calorie = 1 000 calories (cal) = 1 kilocalorie (kcal) = 4 200 joules (J) = 4.2
    kilojoules (kJ)
1 kilojoule = 1 000 J = 240 cal = 0.24 kcal = 0.24 Calories

---

[1] Approximate values given for easy calculation.

GLOSSARY OF VERNACULAR WORDS

Vernacular [1]	Translation
baraza	farmers' meeting
chumvi	salt
dagaa	small fish (Tanzania)
dona	lightly milled maize meal
fufu	boiled, mashed food made from cassava flour
injera	type of baked pancake
irio	traditional Kikuyu food (maize, beans, potatoes, green leaves)
isyo	traditional Kamba food (whole-kernel maize, beans, vegetables)
kapenta	small fish (Zambia)
karanga	groundnut (*Arachis hypogoea*)
kinu	mortar
mafuta	oil
manaragwe	bean
mahindi	maize (grain)
matunda	fruit
mayai	egg
maziwa	milk
mboga	vegetable
mbuyu	baobab
mchi	pestle
mpunga	paddy, unhusked rice
mtama	sorghum, Guinea corn, durra (*Sorghum vulgare*)
muhogo	cassava
nyama	meat
nyoyo	boiled maize
pombe	unfermented sweet beer
samaki	fish
sembe	finely milled maize meal
shamba	farm
togwa	non-alcoholic beverage (= *pombe*)
ugali	stiff porridge made from cereal or cassava flour
ujamaa	cooperative action toward self-sufficiency
uji	thin gruel
ulezi	finger millet (*Eleusine coracana*)
uwele	bulrush millet (*Pennisetum typhoideum*)

---

[1] Mostly Kiswahili.

279

BIBLIOGRAPHY

Cited

DAVIDSON, S., PASSMORE, R., BROCK, J. & TRUSWELL, A.S. *Human nutrition and*
1972   *dietetics*. 6th ed. London, Churchill Livingstone.

FAO.   *Man's right to freedom from hunger, Special Assembly held at FAO, Rome,*
1963   *14 March 1963*. Rome.

FAO.   *Food composition table for use in Africa*. Rome.
1968

FAO.   *Amino-acid content of foods and biological data on proteins*. Rome. FAO
1970   Nutritional Studies No. 24.

FAO.   *Planning and evaluation of applied nutrition programmes*, by M.C. Latham.
1972   Rome. FAO Food and Nutrition Studies No. 26.

FAO.   *Energy and protein requirements: report of a Joint FAO/WHO ad hoc Expert*
1973   *Committee*. Rome. FAO Food and Nutrition Series No. 7.

FAO.   *Handbook on human nutritional requirements*. Rome. FAO Nutritional
1974   Studies No. 28.

FAO.   *Food and nutrition strategies in national development: ninth report of the Joint*
1976   *FAO/WHO Expert Committee on Nutrition*. Rome. FAO Food and Nu-
        trition Series No. 5.

FAO.   Enrichment of dried skim milk. *Food and Nutrition (FAO)*, 3(1): 2-7, Rome.
1977   FAO.

GOMEZ, F., RAMOS GALVAN, R., FRENK, S., CRAVIOTO, J., CHAVEZ, R. & VAZQUEZ, J.
1956   Mortality in second and third degree malnutrition. *J. tropical Pediatrics*,
        2: 77-83.

GOODHART, R.S. & SHILS, M.E. *Modern nutrition in health and disease*. 5th ed.
1973   Philadelphia, Lea and Fabiger.

LATHAM, M.C. Nutrition and infection in national development. *Science*, 188,
1975   561-565.

NICHOLSS, L. *Tropical nutrition and dietetics*. 4th ed. (revised by H.M. Sinclair
1961   and D.B. Jelliffe), London, Baillière, Tindall and Cox.

PLATT, B.S. *Tables of representative values of foods commonly used in tropical*
1962   *countries*. London. HMSO, Medical Research Council. Special Report
        Series No. 302.

STUART, H.C. & STEVENSON, S.S. Physical growth and development. In: NELSON,
1959   W., ed., *Textbook of pediatrics*. 7th ed. Philadelphia, Saunders, p. 12-61.

TANNER, A. & WHITEHOUSE, J. Standards for subcutaneous fat in British children.
1962   *British Medical Journal*, 1.

TROWELL, H.C., DAVIES, J.N.P. & DEAN, R.F.A. *Kwashiorkor*. London, Arnold.
1954

TROWELL, H.C. & JELLIFFE, D.B. *Diseases of children in the subtropics and tropics*.
1958   London, Arnold.

WHO.   *Endemic goitre*. Geneva. WHO Monograph Series No. 44.
1960

WHO.   *The assessment of the nutritional status of a community*, by D.B. Jelliffe.
1966   Geneva. WHO Monograph Series No. 53.

280

WHO. *Manual on public health nutrition*, by K.V. Bailey. Brazzaville, WHO Re-
1975 gional Office for Africa. Document AFR/NUT/79.
WHO. *Vitamin A deficiency and xerophthalmia.* Report of a joint WHO/USAID
1976 meeting. Geneva. Technical Report Series No. 590.
WHO. *A growth chart for international use in maternal and child health care.* Geneva.
1978

Further reading

AMANN, V.F., BELSHAW, D.G.R. & STANFIELD, J.P. (eds.). *Nutrition and food in an*
1972 *African economy.* Kampala, Uganda, Makerere University. 2 vols.
BERG, A. *The nutrition factor.* Washington, The Brookings Institution.
1973
BROWN, L.R. *By bread alone.* New York, Prager.
1974
BURGESS, A. & DEAN, R.F.A. *Malnutrition and food habits.* London, Tavistock.
1962
FAO. *Food and nutrition procedures in times of disaster*, by G.B. Masefield. Rome.
1967 FAO Nutritional Studies No. 21.
FAO. *Learning better nutrition: a second study of approaches and techniques*, by
1967 J.A.S. Ritchie. Rome. FAO Nutritional Studies No. 20
FAO. *Food composition table for use in East Asia.* Rome.
1972
HARDIN, C.M. *Overcoming world hunger.* London, Prentice Hall.
1969
KING, M. (ed.). *Medical care in developing countries.* Oxford, Oxford University
1966 Press.
KING, M., KING, F. & SOEBAGYO MARTODIPOERO. *Primary child care.* Oxford,
1978 Oxford University Press (English language edition); Geneva, WHO (all
other editions).
LATHAM, M.C., MCGANDY, R.B., MCCANN, M.S. & STARE, F.J. *Scope manual*
1970 *on nutrition.* 2nd ed. Kalamazoo, Upjohn.
MCLAREN, D.S. *Nutrition and its disorders.* Edinburgh, Churchill Livingstone.
1972
MCLAREN, D.S. & BURMAN, D. (eds.). *Textbook of paediatric nutrition.* Edinburgh,
1976 Churchill Livingstone.
MORLEY, D. *Paediatric priorities in developing countries.* London, Butterworths.
1973
SCRIMSHAW, N.S. & BEHAR, M. (eds.). *Nutrition and agricultural development.* New
1976 York, Plenum.
WHO. *Infant nutrition in the subtropics and tropics*, by D.B. Jelliffe. Geneva.
1955
WHO. *Interactions of nutrition and infection*, by N.S. Scrimshaw, C.E. Taylor &
1968 J.E. Gordon. Geneva. WHO Monograph Series No. 57.
WHO. *Nutrition in preventive medicine*, by G.H. Beaton & J.M. Bengoa. Geneva.
1976 WHO Monograph Series No. 62.

INDEX

Note: The **bold** figures are main references.

D

Dagaa 68, 186
Day care centre 237
Dementia 99, 102
Dermatitis 99, 100
Dermatosis 117, 127
Dental caries 72, 73, 155
Diabetes 93
Diarrhoea 7, 48, 91, 96, 99, 102, 114, 117, 127, 138, 139
Dietary surveys 32-34
Disaccharide 59, 189
Dysentery 49, 77, 78, 119
Dyspnoea 95, 96, 97
Dyssebacea 151

E

ECG 97
Education 211-214, 218-219
Eggs 19, 64, **188**, 220, 232
Endosperm 162, 163, 166
Enzyme 7, 59, 82, 148

F

Family feeding 226-231
Family planning 15, 16
FAO 2, 64, 113, 280, 281
Fats 54, 55, **60-62**, 150, **193-195**
Fatty acids 61, 62, 193
Ferrous sulfate 38
Fish 71, 186, 220, 234, 246, 247
Fishponds 53, 186, 187, 207, 220
Fluorine (-ide) 66, **72-74**, 155, 160, 196, 209, 210, 222
Foetus 37, 114
Folic acid 85, 144, 145
Follicular hyperkeratosis 150-151
Food fortification 207-209
Food habits - See Taboos
Food and nutrition policy 197-207
Food preservation 11, 78, 83, 222, 245-248
Foods, supplementary 210
Fructose 59
Fruit 183-184, 222, 227, 236, 248

G

Galactose 59
Gastrointestinal infection 7, 42
Ghee 194
Glossitis 154
Glucose 59

Glycogen 59, 60, 63

Glycogen 59, 60, 63
Goats 19, 68, 190, 220
Goitre 71, 72, **139-144**
Gomez classification 131
Groundnuts 64, **177-179**, 193, 194, 234
Guinea pigs 52, 220

H

Haemoglobin **30**, 40, 69, 119, 145
Haemorrhage 86, 111
Heart 71, 95
Height **25-29**, 128
Hepatomegaly 118
Honey 175
Hookworm 6, 31, 49, 71, 119, 121, 130, 144, 146
Hormones 66, 91, 140
Hospital feeding 241

I

Insecticides 221
Insects 18, 185, 221
Iodine 54, 66, 71-72, 140-144, 159, 208
Iodization 144, 222
Iron 38, 47, 54, 66, **69-71**, 144-147, 160, 249

K

Kapenta 68
Keratomalacia 77, **103-106**, 153
Kwashiorkor 7, 8, **113-122**, 128-130, 174

L

Lactation 39, 42, 46, 58, 65
Lactose 59, 189
Lathyrism 149
Legislation 46, 94, 98, 103, 144, 165, 219
Legumes 18, 48, 51, 64, **175-179**, 227
Leprosy 96
Lettuce 18
Liver 63, 70, 71, 79, 83, 185, 186, 233
Locusts 22, 186

M

Magnesium 54, 66
Maize 20, 64, 77, 94, 98-103, 161, 163, **165**
Malaria 6, 31, 119, 130
Maltose 59

285

Sulphonamides 126
Sulphur 54, 62, 66
Sunflower 180
Sweet potatoes 77, 173, 182

T

Taboo 19-20, 22, 188, 219
Tapeworm 84
Tallquist scale 30, 147
Taro 173
Tea 73, 195
Teff 161, 171
Testa 162
Tetany 67, 107, 110
Thiamine - See Vitamin B_1
Thyroid 66, 71, 139-144
Toddler mortality rate 34-35
Togwa 18
Tomato 182
Tryptophan 63, 64, 83, 99, 165, 178
Tsetse fly 10
Tuberculosis 6, 119, 126

U

Ulcer 92, 130, 155
UNICEF 25

V

Vegetable 112, 181-183, 227, 233
Vegetable mixtures 64, 219, 227, **229-231**
Vital statistics 34-35

Vitamins
General 55, **75-89**, 93
A 39, **75-79**, 103-106, 151, 157-158, 193
B group **79-85**, 161, 167, 176
B_1 **79-81**, 93-98, 159, 165
B_2 **81-82**, 94, 129, 155, 158
B_{12} **83-85**, 145
C 21, **86-88**, 107, 111, 112, 161, 172, 180-183, 228, 250
D 69, **88-89**, 106-109, 159, 193
E 75
H 75
K 75
Vomiting 96, 114, 121, 123

W

Wasting 95, 96, 115, 127, 128
Weaning 47-49
Weight **25**, 28, 37, 48, 57, 92, 128, 249
Wernickes' encephalopathy 148
Wheat 20, 161, **168**
WHO 69, 113, 131, 280, 281
Whooping cough 5, 134

X

Xerophthalmia 77, 104, 118
Xerosis 118, **149-150**
X-ray 108, 110, 112

Y

Yams 20, **173**

FAO SALES AGENTS AND BOOKSELLERS

Algeria	Société nationale d'édition et de diffusion, 3, boulevard Zirout-Youcef, Algiers.
Antilles, Netherlands	St. Augustinus Boekhandel, Abraham de Veerstraat 12, Willemstad, Curaçao.
Argentina	Editorial Hemisferio Sur S.R.L., Librería Agropecuaria, Pasteur 743, Buenos Aires.
Australia	Hunter Publications, 58A Gipps Street, Collingwood, Vic. 3066; The Assistant Director, Sales and Distribution, Australian Government Publishing Service, P.O. Box 84, Canberra, A.C.T. 2600, and Australian Government Publications and Inquiry Centres in Canberra, Melbourne, Sydney, Perth, Adelaide and Hobart.
Austria	Gerold & Co., Buchhandlung und Verlag, Graben 31, 1011 Vienna.
Bangladesh	Agricultural Development Agencies in Bangladesh, P.O. Box 5045, Dacca 5.
Belgium	Service des publications de la FAO, M.J. De Lannoy, 202, avenue du Roi, 1060 Brussels. CCP 000-0808993-13.
Belize	The Belize Bookshop, P.O. Box 147, Belize.
Bolivia	Los Amigos del Libro, Perú 3712, Casilla 450, Cochabamba; Mercado 1315, La Paz; René Moreno 26, Santa Cruz; Junín esq. 6 de Octubre, Oruro.
Brazil	Livraria Mestre Jou, Rua Guaipá 518, São Paulo 10; Rua Senador Dantas 19-S205/206, Rio de Janeiro; PRODIL, Promoção e Dist. de Livros Ltda., Av. Venáncio Aires 196, Caixa Postal 4005, Porto Alegre, RS; Livraria Dom Bosco, Rua 14 de Julho 2818, Caixa Postal 962, Campo Grande, MT; A NOSSA LIVRARIA, CLS 103, Bloco C, Lojas 2/6, Brasilia, D.F.; FIMAC, Distribuidora de Livros Ltda., Rua de Bahia 478, Loja 10, Belo Horizonte, ME; METRO CUBICO, Livros e Revistas Técnicas Ltda., Praça São Sebastião, Rua 10 de Julho 613, Caixa Postal 199, Manaus, Amazonas; Distribuidora Luso Mercantil, Rua 13 de Maio 524, Caixa Postal 1124, Belém, Pará; G. Lisbóa Livros Ltda., Rua Princesa Isabel 129, Recife, PE; Livraria Cometa Distribuidora Ltda., Rua da Independencia 46, Salvador, Bahia.
Canada	Renouf Publishing Co. Ltd., 2182 Catherine St. West, Montreal, Que. H3H 1M7.
Chile	Tecnolibro S.A., Merced 753, entrepiso 15, Santiago.
China	China National Publications Import Corporation, P.O. Box 88, Peking.
Colombia	Litexsa Colombiana Ltda., Calle 55, N° 16-44, Apartado Aéreo 51340, Bogotá.
Costa Rica	Librería, Imprenta y Litografía Lehmann S.A., Apartado 10011, San José.
Cuba	Empresa de Comercio Exterior de Publicaciones, O'Reilley 407, Havana.
Cyprus	MAM, P.O. Box 1722, Nicosia.
Denmark	Ejnar Munksgaard, Norregade 6, Copenhagen S.
Dominican Rep.	Fundación Dominicana de Desarrollo, Casa de las Gárgolas, Mercedes 4, Santo Domingo.
Ecuador	Su Librería Cía. Ltda., García Moreno 1172, Apartado 2556, Quito; Calle Chimborazo 416, Guayaquil.
El Salvador	Librería Cultural Salvadoreña S.A., Calle Arce 423, Apartado Postal 2296, San Salvador.
Finland	Akateeminen Kirjakauppa, 1 Keskuskatu, Helsinki.
France	Editions A. Pedone, 13, rue Soufflot, 75005 Paris.
Germany, F.R.	Alexander Horn Internationale Buchhandlung, Spiegelgasse 9, Postfach 3340, Wiesbaden.
Ghana	Fides Enterprises, P.O. Box 1628, Accra; Ghana Publishing Corporation, P.O. Box 3632, Accra.
Greece	''Eleftheroudakis'', 4 Nikis Street, Athens.
Guatemala	Distribuciones Culturales y Técnicas « Artemis », Quinta Avenida 12-11, Zona 1, Guatemala City.
Guinea-Bissau	Conselho Nacional da Cultura, Avenida da Unidade Africana, C.P. 294, Bissau.
Guyana	Guyana National Trading Corporation Ltd., 45-47 Water Street, Georgetown.
Haiti	Max Bouchereau, Librairie « A la Caravelle », B.P. 111, Port-au-Prince.
Honduras	The Bookstore, Apartado Postal 167-C, Tegucigalpa.
Hong Kong	Swindon Book Co., 13-15 Lock Road, Kowloon.
Iceland	Snaebjörn Jónsson and Co. h.f., Hafnarstraeti 9, P.O. Box 1131, Reykjavik.
India	Oxford Book and Stationery Co., Scindia House, New Delhi; 17 Park Street, Calcutta.
Indonesia	P.T. Gunung Agung, 6, Kwitang, Djakarta.
Iran	Iran Book Co. Ltd., 127 Nadershah Avenue, P.O. Box 14-1532, Tehran.
Iraq	National House of Publishing, Distributing and Advertising, Rashid Street, Baghdad.
Ireland	The Controller, Stationery Office, Dublin.
Israel	Emanuel Brown, P.O. Box 4101, 35 Allenby Road and Nachlat Benyamin Street, Tel Aviv; 9 Shlomzion Hamalka Street, Jerusalem.
Italy	Distribution and Sales Section, Food and Agriculture Organization of the United Nations, Via delle Terme di Caracalla, 00100 Rome; Libreria Scientifica Dott. L. De Biasio "Aeiou", Via Meravigli 16, 20123 Milan; Libreria Commissionaria Sansoni "Licosa", Via Lamarmora 45, C.P. 552, 50121 Florence.

FAO SALES AGENTS AND BOOKSELLERS

Jamaica	Teacher Book Centre Ltd., 95 Church Street, Kingston.
Japan	Maruzen Company Ltd., P.O., Box 5050, Tokyo Central 100-31.
Kenya	Text Book Centre Ltd., P.O. Box 47540, Nairobi.
Korea, Rep. of	The Eul-Yoo Publishing Co. Ltd., 5 2-Ka, Chong-ro, Seoul.
Kuwait	Saeed & Samir Bookstore Co. Ltd., P.O. Box 5445, Kuwait.
Luxembourg	Service des publications de la FAO, M.J. De Lannoy, 202, avenue du Roi, 1060 Brussels (Belgium)
Mauritius	Nalanda Company Limited, 30 Bourbon Street, Port Louis.
Mexico	Dilitsa S.A., Puebla 182-D, Apartado 24-448, Mexico City 7, D.F.
Morocco	Librairie « Aux Belles Images », 281, avenue Mohammed V, Rabat.
Netherlands	N.V. Martinus Nijhoff, Lange Voorhout 9, The Hague.
New Zealand	Government Printing Office: Government Bookshops at Rutland Street, P.O. Box 5344, Auckland; Alma Street, P.O. Box 857, Hamilton; Mulgrave Street, Private Bag, Wellington; 130 Oxford Terrace, P.O. Box 1721, Christchurch; Princes Street, P.O. Box 1104, Dunedin.
Nicaragua	Librería Interamericana Nicaragüense S.A., Apartado 2206, Managua.
Nigeria	University Bookshop (Nigeria) Ltd., University of Ibadan, Ibadan.
Norway	ohan Grundt Tanum Bokhandel, Karl Johansgt. GT 41-43, Oslo 1.
Pakistan	Mirza Book Agency, 65 The Mall, Lahore 3.
Panama	Distribuidora Lewis S.A., Edificio Dorasol, Calle 25 y Avenida Balboa, Apartado 1634, Panama 1.
Paraguay	Agencia de Librerías Nizza S.A., Paraguarí 144, Asunción.
Peru	Librería Distribuidora Santa Rosa, Jirón Apurímac 375, Casilla 4937, Lima.
Philippines	The Modern Book Book Company, 928 Rizal Avenue, Manila.
Poland	Ars Polona-Ruch, Krakowskie Przedmiescie 7, Warsaw.
Portugal	Livraria Bertrand, S.A.R.L., Apartado 37, Amadora; Livraria Portugal, Dias y Andrade Ltda., Apartado 2681, Rua do Carmo 70-74, Lisbon-2; Ediçôes ITAU, Avda. República 46A c/v-E, Lisbon-1.
Romania	Ilexim, Calea Grivitei N° 64-66, B.P. 2001, Bucarest.
Saudi Arabia	University Bookshop, Airport Road, P.O. Box 394, Riyadh.
Senegal	Librairie Africa, 58, avenue Georges Pompidou, B.P. 1240, Dakar.
Somalia	"Samater's", P.O. Box 936, Mogadishu.
Spain	Mundi Prensa Libros S.A., Castelló 37, Madrid-1; Librería Agrícola, Fernando VI 2, Madrid-4.
Sri Lanka	M.D. Gunasena and Co. Ltd., 217 Norris Road, Colombo 11.
Suriname	VACO nv in Suriname, P.O. Box 1841, Domineenstraat 26/32, Paramaribo.
Sweden	C.E. Fritzes Kungl. Hovbokhandel, Fredsgatan 2, 103 27 Stockholm 16.
Switzerland	Librairie Payot S.A., Lausanne et Genève; Buchhandlung und Antiquariat, Heinimann & Co., Kirchgasse 17, 8001 Zurich.
Tanzania	Dar es-Salaam Bookshop, P.O. Box 9030, Dar es-Salaam.
Thailand	Suksapan Panit, Mansion 9, Rajadamnern Avenue, Bangkok.
Togo	Librairie du Bon Pasteur, B.P. 1164, Lomé.
Trinidad and Tobago	The Book Shop, 111 Frederick Street, Port of Spain.
Tunisia	Société tunisienne de diffusion, 5, avenue de Carthage, Tunis.
Turkey	Güven Bookstores, Güven Bldg., P.O. Box 145, Müdafaa Cad. 12/5, Kizilay-Ankara; Güven Ari Bookstores, Ankara Cad. No. 45, Cağaloğlu-Istanbul; Güven Bookstore, S.S.K. Konak Tesisleri P-18, Konak-Izmir.
United Kingdom	Her Majesty's Stationery Office, 49 High Holborn, London WC1V 6HB (callers only); P.O. Box 569, London SE1 9NH (trade and London area mail orders); 13a Castle Street, Edinburgh EH2 3AR; 41 The Hayes, Cardiff CF1 1JW; 80 Chichester Street, Belfast BT1 4JY; Brazennose Street, Manchester M60 8AS; 258 Broad Street, Birmingham B1 2HE; Southey House, Wine Street, Bristol BS1 2BQ.
United States of America	UNIPUB, 345 Park Avenue South, New York, N.Y. 10010; mailing address: P.O. Box 433, Murray Hill Station, New York, N.Y. 10016.
Uruguay	Librería Editorial Juan Angel Peri, Alzaibar 1328, Casilla de Correos 1755, Montevideo.
Venezuela	Blume Distribuidora S.A., Av. Rómulo Gallegos esq. 2a. Avenida, Centro Residencial « Los Almendros », Torre 3, Mezzanina, Ofc. 6, Urbanización Montecristo, Caracas.
Yugoslavia	Jugoslovenska Knjiga, Terazije 27/11, Belgrade; Cankarjeva Zalozba, P.O. Box 201-IV, Ljubljana; Prosveta Terazije 16, P.O. Box 555, 11001 Belgrade.
Other countries	Requests from countries where sales agents have not yet been appointed may be sent to: Distribution and Sales Section, Food and Agriculture Organization of the United Nations, Via delle Terme di Caracalla, 00100 Rome, Italy.